CH

The Survival Guide

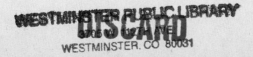

ANGELO ACQUISTA, M.D.

The Survival Guide:
What to Do in a Biological, Chemical, or Nuclear Emergency

RANDOM HOUSE TRADE PAPERBACKS
NEW YORK

A Random House Trade Paperback Original

Copyright © 2003 by Angelo Acquista, M.D., and The Ascent Group, L.L.C.

All rights reserved under International and Pan-American Copyright Conventions. Published in the United States by Random House Trade Paperbacks, a division of Random House, Inc., New York, and simultaneously in Canada by Random House of Canada Limited, Toronto.

RANDOM HOUSE TRADE PAPERBACKS and colophon are trademarks of Random House, Inc.

Library of Congress Cataloging-in-Publication Data

Acquista, Angelo.
　　The survival guide: what to do in a biological, chemical, or nuclear emergency/by Angelo Acquista.
　　　　p. cm.
　　Includes index.
　　ISBN 0-8129-6954-5
　　　　1. Weapons of mass destruction—Health aspects. 2. Terrorism—Health aspects. 3. Disaster medicine. 4. Medical emergencies. I. Title

RC88.9.T47A28 2003　613.6'9—dc21　20022037117

Random House website address: www.atrandom.com

Printed in the United States of America

10 9 8 7 6 5 4 3 2 1

Book design by Cyndi Pena at The Ascent Group

Foreword

We are in a war against terrorists who are well organized, well funded, global, and have access to weapons of mass destruction. As this book will describe, these weapons may be in biological, chemical, nuclear, or radiological form. There is ample evidence that terrorist groups and rogue states are attempting to obtain and develop all of these, and thus it is a time to beware. In the United States, September 11, 2001, not only represented the capability of one particular terrorist network, but it also horrifically revealed the unrestrained, savage intent that can exist in those who promote terrorism.

There is a major distinction among terrorists. The first kind swears to a cause, such as righting a perceived injustice or advancing a political or secessionist goal, that they are dedicated to publicizing in an effort to win support. These terrorists attempt to advance their cause with sporadic acts of sensationalistic violence that will bring the desired media attention they believe is so critical to furthering their objective. While not averse to sacrificing innocent people, they are generally somewhat constrained by the desire not to alienate the very audience they hope someday to win over.

The second type, religious terrorists, are consumed by radical motivations that do not distinguish between perceived combatants and others. The ultimate terror is that for these people all boundaries, geographic and human, are absent. Their only goal is to rid the world of those they have decreed unfit to live or whom they believe oppose their way of thinking; they believe it is a divine imperative and are acting on "God's orders." As such, they make no distinction between enemies and innocent men, women, and children. Their desire is simple: to kill as many "infidels" as possible.

Unfortunately, all types of organized terrorism have been going on for hundreds of years, and they are now, alarmingly, building with a steady momentum. It is only the shocking awareness caused by 9/11 that is recent. As a result, our response to terrorism has only recently become serious, despite attacks on American interests overseas, such as the U.S. Embassy bombings in Kenya and Tanzania in 1998, and on our homeland, such as the truck bombing of the World Trade Center in 1993. In hindsight, we now recognize these attacks as stark warnings. America—and most of the Westernized world—are obviously targets for terrorists.

Government spending for finding and disrupting terrorist organizations that target the United States and U.S. interests has dramatically increased, but we are only in the beginning stages of our mission. For example, legislation to give the FBI more ability to monitor terrorists was passed by Congress and signed into law by President Clinton in 1994, but only after 9/11 was it implemented. Furthermore, the Department of

Homeland Security has only just been created, and the many actions it will take to protect our country are just now being undertaken. In certain areas, like port security, we still have a long way to go.

As well as paying attention to organized terrorist regimes, however, we should not forget that random acts of terrorism can easily reach the scope of organized terrorists' most intricate plots. It only took some bags of fertilizer and diesel fuel, a high school education, and a U-Haul truck to bring down half of the Alfred P. Murrah Federal Building in Oklahoma City in 1995. With the wide availability of information, especially over the Internet, we need to be prepared to deal not only with organized terror networks but also with everything from copycat terrorists to the outraged, laid-off employee who learns how to aerosolize a biologic agent from published procedures.

Awareness, preparation, and effective rapid response to terrorist acts are critical at all levels of our society, not only for those who will be there in the aftermath—the police, fire departments, paramedics, other emergency service staff, and hospital personnel—but for the people who will truly be first on the scene: ordinary citizens. You may be the one who identifies the symptoms or knows what to do during a biological, chemical, or radiological incident based upon what you've read in this book. *The Survival Guide* is an invaluable tool for helping everyone in our society to become better aware of potential threats and to better carry out our role.

Armed with only information, you could save your life and those of others. The fight against terrorism has become the responsibility of all of us, and there is no weapon more effective than information.

James K. Kallstrom
Senior Advisor for Counter-Terrorism
Office of the Governor
State of New York

Table of Contents

Introduction

My background in pulmonary and tropical diseases brought me to New York City's Office of Emergency Management (OEM) in 1999, where I have served as their pro bono medical director. In May 2001, I sat in a conference room on the twenty-third floor of the World Trade Center Plaza's building number seven, where OEM was housed, with Mayor Rudolph Giuliani and representatives of federal, state, and city emergency and health agencies. We were there to discuss an immense and terrifying problem: hundreds of people in the city of New York were suddenly falling ill and dying from a virulent and fast-acting disease, and no one knew why. The city was convulsed with panic.

Mayor Giuliani spent much of the meeting outlining a strategy to help the various agencies—such as the Federal Emergency Management Agency, the state health department, or the city police department—to reach out to, calm, and treat afflicted and fearful New Yorkers. I sat watching the anxious faces of the people sitting around the table with me, searching with them for answers to endless difficult questions. I had never seen an outbreak like this in my career. New York's Syndromic Surveillance System (composed of various elements that help detect biological events, such as disease-reporting requirements for healthcare workers) had identified an unusually high number of patients with a flulike illness who, within five to seven days, were developing pneumonia and dying, predominantly on the Upper East Side of Manhattan. I could think of no disease fitting this description of rapid deterioration that might be expected in this part of the city, or country, for that matter. As each hour passed, we were told that more people were falling ill and dying, and that the disease had spread across New York City. We then learned that all of the patients had attended a basketball game at the Lexington Avenue Armory two weeks earlier. When the blood cultures of patients revealed *Yersinia pestis,* the bacteria that causes plague, we became certain that there must have been a deliberate aerosol release of the bacteria, especially since there are normally only about a dozen plague cases reported in the United States every year, and those are generally in the western states. Immediately we discussed enforcing a quarantine for infected victims and for the city itself, which would involve shutting down all transportation in and out of the five boroughs of New York City, closing bridges, tunnels, railroads, and airports. We then talked about issues like how the police would manage the quarantine, how antibiotics would be distributed to the millions of residents, who should receive priority treatment, who should receive prophylaxis, and how the hospital system would care for a major metropolitan city infected with this highly contagious disease. There was so much to address, and time was running out.

Luckily, for everyone in the room and in the city, the entire scenario was a fabrication; it was the Office of Emergency Management's Operation REDEX (Recognition, Evaluation, and Decision-making Exercise). Attempting to educate and prepare city officials for a biological terrorist attack, OEM had coordinated the event and organized a number of test situations for dealing with an outbreak of pneumonic plague and other deadly disease candidates. After this exercise was concluded, another scenario—unnamed, so that everyone on the case would work through it as an actual event with all of its idiosyncrasies—was scheduled for September 12, 2001.

But our plans were changed. Today, building number seven, where we had that first meeting, is gone, destroyed with the twin towers on September 11—and with much of the sense of security that was once part of life in New York City and in the rest of the country. And a month later, as if that were not disturbing enough, anthrax was delivered in the mail to New York City offices, just the sort of attack we had hypothetically dealt with. I was asked to serve on the Mayoral Advisory Task Force for Bioterrorism that Mayor Giuliani assembled in response to this new and now very real threat. The objective of this task force, similar in some ways to that of the May mock scenario, was to review the syndromic surveillance systems and to consider citywide antibiotic issues relating to bacterial sensitivities, preventive medical tactics, therapeutic recommendations, and drug dispensing. We also focused on the availability of rapid diagnostic technology for microorganism and disease identification and on implementing a plan for medical community awareness, including physician education.

I realized that, in addition to lending my expertise as a physician, I could share with the public the valuable information we collected in our meetings before September 11, along with the wisdom we gained from having to deal so unexpectedly with the anthrax attacks. However, though the anthrax scare of October 2001 brought bioweapon threats to the forefront, they are certainly not our only risk. In fact, many chemical weapons are much easier and cheaper to produce. Moreover, many believe that radiological weapons are the most probable choice of terrorists. *The Survival Guide* was thus created to cover a broad scope of potential terrorism threats.

The word *terrorism* is derived from the Latin word for fear and was originally used in 1793 to describe government by intimidation during the French Reign of Terror. Because the key mechanism that allows terrorists of any kind to attain profound effects is fear, removing this element is an integral weapon in combating terrorism. As it is human nature to be afraid of the unknown, much of the fear of terrorism in the modern age—

biological, chemical, and nuclear attacks—is based upon ignorance. In the course of researching and writing this book, many of my own personal fears regarding these weapons have been greatly reduced. Knowledge is essential not only for alleviating our worries and allowing us to be prepared, but also for minimizing panic and ensuring the best possible outcome by giving us effective steps to follow during and after an attack.

There is no other book that provides detailed, easy-to-find, easy-to-read information for the layperson regarding an extensive range of atomic, biological, and chemical weapons of mass destruction, and so this book is written for you. Terrorists wish most to make us afraid; we can empower ourselves with the knowledge offered here.

Angelo Acquista, M.D.

HOW TO USE THIS BOOK

Each biological, chemical, and nuclear chapter in this book includes some or all of the following sections. Please take a moment to read their descriptions, as we describe here which recommendations are meant for trained professionals and which are meant for the ordinary citizen during the course and aftermath of an incident.

WHAT IT IS: A description of the biological, chemical, or nuclear agent.

WHAT IT DOES: A description of what the agent does to the human body.

HOW YOU CATCH IT / HOW YOU GET EXPOSED: This section describes how you would acquire the illness, such as how it is absorbed and whether it is spread from person to person.

HOW DO YOU TELL WHAT IT IS?: Since chemicals often have immediate effects, this section in the chemical weapons chapters deals with indicators that may help identify the agent, such as smell. It should be remembered that descriptions are for pure chemicals or their most common mixtures; if chemicals are blended with other substances, their characteristics can change.

ASSESSMENT OF RISK: This section assesses the risk to U.S. residents that a particular agent might be used and the degree of danger it holds if it were used.

Centers for Disease Control Ratings: The Centers for Disease Control has rated potential bioterrorism threats from A (top priority) to C (the lowest priority), following these general areas as criteria: (1) public-health impact based on illness and death; (2) delivery potential to large populations based on stability of the agent, ability to mass-produce and distribute a virulent agent, and potential for person-to-person transmission of the agent; (3) public perception as related to public fear and potential civil disruption; and (4) special public-health preparedness needs based on stockpile requirements, enhanced surveillance, and diagnostic needs.

CDC Rating	Priority	What the Rating Means
Category A	Highest priority	These biological agents include organisms that pose a risk to national security because they: - Can be easily spread, especially person to person - Result in high mortality rates and have the potential for major public-health impact - Might cause public panic and social disruption - Require special action for public-health preparedness
Category B	Second-highest priority	These agents include those that: - Are moderately easy to disseminate - Result in moderate rate of disease and low mortality rates - Require specific enhancements of the CDC's diagnostic capacity and disease surveillance
Category C	Third-highest priority	These are biological agents currently not believed to present a high bioterrorism risk to public health but that could emerge as future threats (as scientific understanding of these agents improves) because of: - Availability - Ease of production and dissemination - Potential for high disease and mortality rates and major health impact

Risk of Use in an Attack: This section deals with the availability, stability, and producibility of the agent and the history of prior use.

How Dangerous Is It?: This assesses what we can expect in terms of how contagious and/or deadly the agent might be in an attack.

TIMELINE OF ILLNESS: This section outlines the normal course of illness: the period from exposure to when symptoms begin (the incubation period) and the expected course of illness or effects over time.

SYMPTOMS: This section describes the major symptoms that may result after exposure to the particular biological, chemical, or nuclear agent. It is important to remember that commonly found symptoms are listed for each scenario, and if affected, you may experience only some, or none, of the symptoms listed. This section is intended for informational purposes only and should not substitute consulting with your doctor if you are concerned you are ill.

EMERGENCY RESPONSE: Suggestions for immediate, emergency response in the event of a particular biological, chemical, or radiological attack are given here. While some information in this book describes what trained professionals will carry out, this section is for everyone. Note that in the presence of emergency personnel, you should follow their instructions.

TESTING AND DIAGNOSIS: This section lists tests that may be performed to confirm either the presence of the agent in the environment or the specific illness in the person. Most of these tests must be performed by trained professionals, such as your doctor, laboratory personnel, or emergency responders.

TREATMENT: This section describes the standard course of treatment for the particular illness caused by the biological, chemical, or radiological agent. It is for informational purposes only; in most cases the decision about when and how to treat should be made by medical professionals.

> **NOTE:** This book is intended to be used only as a reference tool for consumers who want more information about biological, chemical, and nuclear emergencies, and about the drugs and treatments their physicians may prescribe for them. It is not meant to replace the professional advice and expertise of your physician, or to encourage patients to evaluate the risks and benefits of using certain medications and treatments without consulting their healthcare providers. Only a physician can choose the best treatment for you, as well as prescribe drugs, advise on their exact dosages and possible drug interactions, and monitor and evaluate the patient's response and reaction to prescription medications.

VACCINE: In biological weapons chapters, this section addresses whether a vaccine exists for prevention and/or treatment of the disease. No vaccines exist for chemical or nuclear agents.

ANTIDOTE: This section, in chemical weapons chapters only, addresses whether an antidote exists for treatment.

CHILDREN: Special precautions for children specific to the chapter are described here. Note that Chapter 31 in the *EMERGENCY PLANNING* section addresses more general concerns and recommendations for children, particularly in relation to emergency planning, coping with terrorism, and their vulnerabilities to biological, chemical, and radiological agents.

PREGNANCY: Special precautions for pregnant women are given in this section.

SPECIAL PRECAUTIONS: This section lists any additional precautions specific to the biological, chemical, or radiological agent.

ENVIRONMENTAL DECONTAMINATION AND CLEANUP: This section describes what generally must be done to decontaminate the environment where a biological, chemical, or radiological incident has taken place. It is for informational purposes only and does not necessarily mean it is safe for the untrained and unprotected to perform. You could put yourself at risk of further exposure to the contaminant during cleanup. In many cases, specialized protective clothing and respiratory protection are required by trained professionals. It is extremely important to listen to emergency officials after an event to determine your specific course of action, which may vary from case to case. For example, you may be directed to wait until professional decontamination personnel come to you or you may be instructed to perform simple, nonhazardous decontamination procedures yourself.

HOW YOU CAN PREPARE: This section recommends actions you might take to prepare for the specific event covered in the chapter.

ADDITIONAL RESOURCES: This section lists resources that may be helpful regarding the specific agent or weapon. Note that the *Public Resources and Contact Information* section of the book may have additional helpful resources; this general, more comprehensive list includes contact information for things like federal and private agencies that assist during biological, chemical, and nuclear emergencies.

U.S. GOVERNMENT EMERGENCY AND SECURITY SUPPORT

Emergency Federal Support Timeline
In general, after a natural or manmade emergency, the U.S. federal government would respond according to the timeline outlined below. For coordinated local, state, and national responses specific to biological, chemical, or radiological/nuclear events, see Chapter 16, *Unidentified Biological Agent*, Chapter 24, *Unidentified Chemical Agent*, and Chapter 29, *Event with Unknown Radioactivity*.

Hours 0–6
Local fire, emergency medical services (EMS), and law enforcement respond; if a disaster is expected to last more than 24 hours, the government must declare a "state of emergency" in order to activate the federal response; the **Office of Emergency Preparedness (OEP)** may intervene; the **Federal Emergency Management Agency (FEMA)** may also be activated.

Hours 6–12
The **Centers for Disease Control (CDC)** may release emergency-supply "push packs" from the **National Pharmaceutical Stockpile (NPS)** within 12 hours; pharmacists, public-health experts, and emergency teams may assist with the distribution and delivery of the push packs; the **Metropolitan Medical Strike Team (MMST)** may be called upon to

coordinate the resources of local, state, and federal emergency response teams; patients, if possible, will be sent to area hospitals that participate in the **Public Health Service's (PHS) National Disaster Medical System (NDMS)**; **Federal Disaster Medical Assistance Teams (DMATs)** will perform some medical care and evacuation services if required.

Hours 12–24

Additional, neighboring MMSTs may be activated upon request and additional supplies may be ordered by the MMST; the **Environmental Protection Agency (EPA)** may be called upon to respond to chemical, radioactive, or biological incidents; push packs may be followed by supplemental materials in Vendor Managed Inventory (VMI) packages.

Hour 36

MMST will be demobilized if no longer needed.

Hour 48 and after

State officials begin collaborating with FEMA for long-term disaster relief if necessary.

The U.S. Department of Homeland Security

On November 25, 2002, President Bush signed into law the Homeland Security Act, thus creating a new department in the U.S. government, the Department of Homeland Security. Its stated mission is to:

- Prevent terrorist attacks within the United States
- Reduce America's vulnerability to terrorism
- Minimize the damage and recover from attacks that occur

To this end, the department is organized into four divisions:

1) Border and Transportation Security

Responsible for securing our nation's borders and transportation systems, managing who and what enters our homeland, and working to prevent the entry of terrorists and the instruments of terrorism, while ensuring the efficient flow of legitimate traffic.

2) Emergency Preparedness and Response

Will ensure the preparedness of our nation's emergency response professionals, provide the federal government's response, and aid America's recovery from terrorist attacks and natural disasters.

3) Chemical, Biological, Radiological, and Nuclear Countermeasures

Will lead the federal government's efforts in preparing for and responding to the full range of terrorist threats involving weapons of mass destruction.

4) Information Analysis and Infrastructure Protection

Will merge under one roof the capability to identify and assess current and future threats to our homeland, map those threats against our current vulnerabilities, inform the president, issue timely warnings, and immediately take or effect appropriate preventive and protective action.

Homeland Security Advisory System Recommendations

Risk of Attack	What It Means and Recommended Actions
GREEN (LOW)	– Low risk of terrorist attack – Be prepared by being informed of what to do before, during, and after various possible attack scenarios, be they bomb blasts or biological, chemical, nuclear, or radiological attacks
BLUE (GUARDED)	– General risk of terrorist attack – Follow recommendations from the green level – Be alert to suspicious activity in your environment, and report it to the proper authorities – Review and update emergency response procedures and supplies – Listen for updates from government officials
YELLOW (ELEVATED)	– Significant risk of terrorist attack – Follow all recommendations from the above levels – Refine protective measures if specific threats are given – Review evacuation plans and alternate routes to and from work and school; have evacuation supplies stocked and in place – Have shelter-in-place supplies stocked and in place
ORANGE (HIGH)	– High risk of terrorist attack – Security efforts with armed forces or law enforcement agencies may be implemented – Follow all recommendations from the above levels – Take additional precautions at public events – Exercise caution when traveling
RED (SEVERE)	– Severe risk of terrorist attack – Emergency response personnel may be assigned, and specially trained teams may be pre-positioned – Transportation systems may be monitored, redirected, or constrained – Public and government facilities may be closed – Follow all recommendations from the above levels – Listen to TV and radio for current information and instructions from public authorities – Adhere to any travel restrictions announced by government officials – Be prepared to evacuate or shelter-in-place if instructed to do so

ANTHRAX

DISEASE
Anthrax

ORGANISM RESPONSIBLE	TYPE
Bacillus anthracis	Bacteria

HOW YOU CATCH IT

Breathing it in, eating contaminated food, and through exposed skin

TIME FROM EXPOSURE TO ILLNESS

INHALATION (BREATHED IN): 1–60 days
INTESTINAL (DIGESTIVE TRACT): 3–7 days
CUTANEOUS (SKIN): 1–2 days

MAJOR SYMPTOMS

INHALATION: Initially very similar to the flu (fever, headache, abdominal pain, vomiting, coughing, chest pain) but without nasal congestion; with increasing and eventually severe respiratory (breathing) difficulties
INTESTINAL: Abdominal pain, bloody diarrhea, fever, nausea, vomiting, sore throat, ulcer at the base of tongue
CUTANEOUS: First an itchy bump forms, which then becomes an ulcer that will eventually scab over

EMERGENCY RESPONSE

AIRBORNE RELEASE:
- Leave area of exposure immediately
- Cover nose and mouth with fabric (wet if possible) or an N95 respiratory mask
- Try to hold your breath until out of the area or take shallow breaths if necessary
- Limit movement, as going from room to room will spread the anthrax spores
- Remove clothes and place them and any items potentially exposed in double-plastic sealed bags
- Wash body thoroughly with copious amounts of soap and hot water
- Wash eyes with saline solution or flush with water
- Early antibiotic treatment is essential for survival

TREATMENT

Antibiotics such as ciprofloxacin and doxycycline

POSSIBILITY OF DEATH

INHALATION: 90–100% (untreated) to 30–50% (treated, depending on how quickly antibiotics are started)
INTESTINAL: 50% (untreated)
CUTANEOUS: 20% (untreated) to very low (treated)

VACCINE

Available through the Centers for Disease Control

WHAT IT IS

Anthrax is a potentially deadly infection caused by the bacteria *Bacillus anthracis*. The bacteria occur naturally in the soil throughout Asia, Africa, Great Britain, parts of Europe, South and Central America, the Caribbean, the Middle East, and some U.S. regions such as in Texas, Oklahoma, and the Mississippi Valley. From 1955–1999, 236 cases of anthrax, most of them skin infections, were reported in the United States. The last case of inhalational anthrax, before October 2001, was in 1976.

The anthrax bacteria usually infect warm-blooded animals, including humans. Although it is rare in the United States and other industrialized nations for animals to carry anthrax, due to vaccination programs, humans usually contract it by coming in contact with infected animals or animal parts, or from contaminated soil. It remains a problem in developing countries.

Living anthrax bacteria can only survive for around 24 hours outside of an animal or person's body. However, when deprived of nutrients the bacterium goes into a resting phase and forms a hardy, protective shell around itself. Called a spore in this phase, it can last for centuries. Spores cannot move around on their own or reproduce, but once inside a living body again, they will come to life and cause an infection.

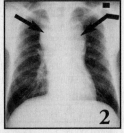

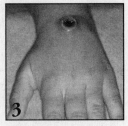

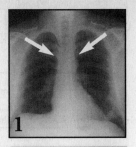

1) Arrows point to the lymph node area (mediastinum) of normal lungs. 2) Arrows point to enlarged lymph nodes and swelling within the chest due to inhalation anthrax. 3) Cutaneous, or skin, anthrax lesion, about 5 days after exposure. The ulcer is enlarged and swollen and the base is turning black.

Infection is caused by the bacterial organisms or spores entering the body through either breathing them in ("INHALATION ANTHRAX"), entering through exposed skin ("CUTANEOUS ANTHRAX"), or through the mouth and digestive track ("GASTROINTESTINAL ANTRHAX"). The type of infection that follows depends on the manner in which the bacteria enter the body.

WHAT IT DOES

INHALATION ANTHRAX: Breathing anthrax spores into the lungs may lead to severe lung damage. The spores become living bacteria once they are inside the body (sometimes even several months later) and start producing toxins, chemicals that damage a cell and can kill it. In inhalation anthrax, the anthrax toxins cause death of lung and lymphatic tissue. Lungs infected with anthrax will fill with blood and fluids, thus preventing oxygen from entering the blood. Once the bacteria are in the lungs, they can get into the blood circulation and spread the disease throughout the body, including the brain (meningitis).

GASTROINTESTINAL ANTHRAX: Open sores form inside the body along the digestive tract, such as in the throat or intestine. Toxins affect the digestive tract first, then can spread to the rest of the body through the circulation.

CUTANEOUS ANTHRAX: Anthrax bacteria release toxins that kill skin cells, which leads to an ulcer (open circular wound) forming and eventually to a black scab of dead skin. It rarely leads to widespread infection.

HOW YOU CATCH IT

INHALATION: Rarely occurs in nature. Contracted by breathing in anthrax spores in the air.
GASTROINTESTINAL: Rarely occurs in nature. Contracted by eating undercooked, contaminated meat, meat products, or dairy products.
CUTANEOUS: Most common. Contracted through exposed skin and cuts and abrasions in the skin, usually by contact with infected animals, animal parts such as fur or bone, or soil containing anthrax spores.

Transmission from Person-to-Person?
No. Theoretically the disease could be contracted by picking up anthrax spores from another person's anthrax skin sores, but an actual case has never been documented.

ASSESSMENT OF RISK

Centers for Disease Control Rating = Highest Priority (Category A)

Risk of Use in an Attack
In the minds of many experts, anthrax represents the single greatest biological warfare threat. The reasons for this are: (1) It can easily be concealed, (2) it is very deadly, (3) it is accessible, (4) it can be stored for decades and is not destroyed by disinfectants or extreme temperatures, and (5) it could be delivered to large populations and cause mass casualties.

As a weapon, anthrax would most likely be sprayed into the air (or "aerosolized"), so it would be acquired by INHALATION. It would be a difficult technical process to make a large enough batch of anthrax that could be aerosolized to affect large numbers of people. In addition, anthrax spores naturally stick to things and clump together, keeping them from staying airborne for very long and also making the clumps too big to get deep into the lungs and cause infection. With the correct, highly specialized laboratory skills and delivery mechanism, however, an aerosolized attack could be achieved. "Weaponized" anthrax means that the anthrax spores have been manipulated to make them easy to use as a weapon, such as designing them to not clump together or making them resistant to drug treatment.

Today, at least 17 nations are believed to have offensive biological weapons programs; it is uncertain how many are working with anthrax.

How Dangerous Is It?
INHALATION: Extremely dangerous. Death can occur in 1–5 days. Death is certain without treatment, and even with treatment begun within the first 2 days may occur in 50–90% of cases.
GASTROINTESTINAL: Death rate is high (50%) if the illness is not properly identified and treated early.
CUTANEOUS: Without antibiotic treatment, death rate could be as high as 20%, but with antibiotic treatment there is a high probability of complete cure (mild sores would heal without scarring).

TIMELINE OF ILLNESS

INHALATION: Time from exposure to illness is usually 1–6 days, but it could be up to 60 days after exposure.
GASTROINTESTINAL: Symptoms begin 3–7 days after exposure, and death can follow within 2–5 days from then.
CUTANEOUS: Time from exposure to illness could be from immediate to 1–2 days.

SYMPTOMS

INHALATION: Initially very similar to a cold or the flu (feeling of tiredness, body aches, headache, mild fever, dry cough, mild chest pain, but no runny nose). There is sometimes a period of 1–3 days after the patient first becomes sick when he or she appears to be getting better. However, after this period the patient rapidly becomes extremely ill. The second stage of infection can result in increasing breathing difficulties, sweating, high fever, vomiting of blood, increased heart rate, and the patient can turn bluish in color.

GASTROINTESTINAL–ABDOMINAL: Resembles a severe case of food poisoning. Loss of appetite, nausea, vomiting of blood, fever, body aches. In later stages, bloody diarrhea, severe stomach pain, and abdominal swelling due to fluids filling that area.

GASTROINTESTINAL–OROPHARYNGEAL: Fever, swelling of the neck, severe sore throat, difficulty swallowing, ulcers at the base of the tongue.

CUTANEOUS: First an itchy bump forms, which turns into a blisterlike sore. The blister breaks and an ulcer (open round wound) forms by the second day. Swelling can occur, as well as mild fever and muscle aches. The ulcer turns black 7–10 days after the first bump forms, and then over a period of 1–2 weeks it will dry out, scab over, and the scab will fall off.

EMERGENCY RESPONSE

INHALATION:

- **Leave area of exposure immediately.**

- **Cover your mouth with wet fabric or an N95 respiratory mask and try to close your eyes and hold your breath** for as long as possible if you are in an area where suspected anthrax is being blown into the air. *The greatest risk of infection is while the spores are in the air.* Take shallow breaths if you have to breathe.

- **Limit movement from room to room,** as this will spread the anthrax spores.

- **Remove clothes and place them and any items potentially exposed in double-plastic sealed bags.** Do not bring inside your home if you are exposed outside the home.

- **Wash body thoroughly** with lots of soap and water, using hot water (155ºF or more) if possible.

- **Wash eyes** with saline solution or flush with water.

- **Early antibiotic treatment is essential for survival.** A delay even by hours may mean the difference between life and death.

- **All persons with fever** or evidence of the disease in an area where anthrax cases are known to be occurring should be treated for anthrax until proven that they are not carrying the bacteria.

- **Persons with high suspicion of infection should be taken to a hospital immediately.**

GASTROINTESTINAL:

- **Begin antibiotic treatment as soon as possible.**

- **Persons with high suspicion of infection should be taken to a hospital immediately.**

CUTANEOUS:

- **Wash body thoroughly** with copious amounts of soap and water. Wash eyes with saline solution or flush with water.
- **Remove clothes and seal in double-plastic bags.**

TESTING AND DIAGNOSIS

Diagnosis

− Aerosolized anthrax would be odorless and invisible following release.

− Diagnosis is made by a combination of symptoms and laboratory test results.

− The sudden appearance in a city or region of a large number of patients with flulike illness and a high fatality rate, with nearly half of all deaths occurring within 24–72 hours from the time that symptoms begin, would suggest a release of inhalation anthrax as a biological weapon.

Testing

Standard testing	- Blood sample taken for culture. Can show growth of anthrax in 6–24 hours if infection is present. - For inhalation infection, chest x-ray can show a distinctive pattern. - For cutaneous anthrax, a sample from the wound fluid may be taken for microscopic analysis and culture.
Rapid testing	Called a polymerase chain reaction (PCR) test, it uses DNA to identify anthrax.
Sampling the inside of the nose	Using a Q-tip-like swab, this test shows only if a person *may* have been exposed. It is not a test to tell if a person has the anthrax infection, as some people who are exposed will never develop an infection.
Atmospheric testing	An atmospheric warning system to detect an aerosol cloud of anthrax has been developed.

TREATMENT

It is crucial to begin anthrax treatment before the bacteria begin producing toxins, which is as soon as the spores "vegetate" into bacteria (anywhere from 1–60 days after entry into the body). These toxins are chemicals that can damage and kill cells. Though antibiotics will kill the bacteria themselves, it is the toxin that does the damage, and there is no drug to stop the toxin. Fortunately, promising antitoxin drugs are currently being developed.

It is also extremely important to follow through to the end the entire course of antibiotics, which could be prescribed for as long as 2–3 months. This is because antibiotics are effective only against live, growing bacteria—not against the spores. Thus, if there are spores left in the body after antibiotic treatment is discontinued, they may vegetate and start up a new infection.

INHALATION:
- **Antibiotics:** There are many antibiotics to choose from that will usually kill anthrax bacteria. Ciprofloxacin ("cipro") and doxycycline are generally the most effective and should be used until it is known whether other antibiotics will work. Other antibiotics that may be considered are rifampin, imipenem, and clindamycin.
- The Centers for Disease Control recommends that at least 2 antibiotics be given for inhalation anthrax. In conjunction with ciprofloxacin or doxycycline, rifampin, vancomycin, penicillin, ampicillin, chloramphenicol, imipenem, clindamycin, or clarithromycin has been suggested.
- A **ventilator** (mechanical breathing machine) may be necessary.

GASTROINTESTINAL: Early **antibiotic treatment** is crucial. For suggested drug therapy, see inhalation anthrax.

CUTANEOUS: **Antibiotics** have not been shown to speed healing of anthrax skin sores but may prevent an infection from spreading to the rest of the body. Ciprofloxacin or doxycycline is usually used.

VACCINE
Effectiveness. An early version of the U.S. vaccine was 93% successful in protecting against the disease. Full treatment involves 6 shots followed by an annual booster.
Getting Vaccinated After Exposure. Vaccination after exposure in an anthrax attack is recommended. It should be supplemented with antibiotics to protect against remaining dormant spores in the body.
Availability. It is currently available only to military personnel and others whose jobs put them at risk for exposure. It is approved for healthy adults between the ages of 18 and 65 only.

CHILDREN
Antibiotics
- A full course of ciprofloxacin treatment is not recommended for children younger than 16–18 years as it could have serious lasting side effects. However, in a known anthrax attack, given the dangers of infection, ciprofloxacin is recommended as the first treatment. If it is found that another antibiotic such as penicillin will work, that should be substituted.

- Doxycycline is usually not recommended for children under 8 years of age. It has been known to cause retarded bone growth and discolored teeth after being given to infants. However, given the deadliness of anthrax infection, it may be recommended by your doctor.

Vaccine
- No studies have been done on the safety of the vaccine in children, but based on studies with other similar vaccines, it is likely it would be safe and effective.

PREGNANCY

Antibiotics
- Fluoroquinolones and doxycycline are usually not recommended during pregnancy. You should discuss their risks with your doctor.
- Ciprofloxacin is considered to be the antibiotic of choice for 60-day preventive treatment (prophylaxis) following inhalational anthrax exposure in symptom-free pregnant women. Studies suggest that ciprofloxacin is safe during pregnancy, but no controlled, long-term human studies have been done. You should discuss the risks of taking ciprofloxacin with your doctor.
- Centers for Disease Control guidelines for treatment of anthrax infection in pregnant women recommend either ciprofloxacin or doxycycline with one or two other antibiotics added for inhalational anthrax or systemic involvement.
- In instances where penicillin has been shown to be effective against the specific strain of anthrax, prophylactic treatment with penicillin or amoxicillin may be considered.
- Ciprofloxacin and other fluoroquinolones, penicillin, and doxycycline are excreted in breast milk. Therefore, a breastfeeding woman should consult her physician for the appropriate antibiotic.

Vaccine
- The vaccine is neither licensed nor recommended for use during pregnancy.

SPECIAL PRECAUTIONS

Even after an apparent cure, and the entire course of antibiotics has been completed, patients should be monitored for 1–2 months post-treatment for signs of the recurrence of anthrax. Seek medical care immediately if you develop symptoms such as fever, malaise, or a cough. Because the spores are so hardy, it is possible they will remain in the body and vegetate at a later time.

Mail Handling
- Avoid holding letters to your nose or sniffing them before opening.

- Don't shake or jostle the contents.
- Open mail slowly with a letter opener rather than with your hands.
- Wash your hands thoroughly after handling mail.
- If an item of unknown origin feels like it contains powder, has a threatening message on it, has excessive postage, has a strange odor, is soiled or oily, or has misspellings of common words, names, or titles, be extra cautious when opening it.
- If an item of mail contains powder of an unknown substance:
  - Do *not* carry the item around—this will spread the anthrax spores.
  - Try to place the item in a sealed plastic bag or container, or cover with a wet cloth, book, magazine, or anything else available to keep the powder from blowing into the air.
  - Leave the room and close the door.
  - Follow decontamination steps in *EMERGENCY RESPONSE* section above.

ENVIRONMENTAL DECONTAMINATION AND CLEANUP

- A number of disinfectants, such as 0.5% sodium hypochlorite solution (1 part household bleach, 9 parts water), are effective in cleaning surfaces contaminated with infected body fluids.
- Alcohol is not sufficient to kill anthrax spores.
- Line drying clothes in the sun would allow ultraviolet (UV) rays to kill anthrax.
- Decontamination of large urban areas would be extremely difficult and probably not necessary.
- In an enclosed building, fumigation with the gas form of chlorine dioxide and the liquid form for surfaces may be used, as it was in the Senate building after the October 2001 anthrax contamination. Afterward, the chemical sodium bisulfite was used to break down the gas. Office equipment and supplies were treated with ethylene oxide (commonly used to sanitize medical instruments).
- Administration of the vaccine would be more practical than environmental cleanup.
- Proper burial or cremation must be undertaken with care to avoid further transmission of spores.

HOW YOU CAN PREPARE

Wash hands regularly. As the majority of all infections are spread this way, adopting this habit will prevent everyday infections as well.

Keep respiratory mask N95 on hand.

Keep health-facility and emergency phone numbers readily available (see *ADDITIONAL RESOURCES* below and the *Public Resources and Contact Information* section of the book). In the event of an attack, antibiotic treatment should begin immediately.

On self-prescribing antibiotics: Unnecessary and frequent use of antibiotics could kill the weakest bacteria and leave the strongest to keep reproducing and infecting others. In this way, we could build antibiotic-resistant bacteria, or bacteria that cannot be killed by common (or possibly any) antibiotics. Furthermore, allergic reactions to antibiotics are not uncommon and can even be life-threatening, and they may also cross-react with other medications you are taking. The U.S. government has antibiotics stockpiled for our nation in the case of an anthrax attack.

ADDITIONAL RESOURCES

American College of Physicians–American Society of Internal Medicine
   www.acponline.org/bioterro/index.html#anthrax
Centers for Disease Control (CDC)
   www.bt.cdc.gov/agent/anthrax/anthraxgen.asp
   www.cdc.gov/ncidod/dbmd/diseaseinfo/anthrax_g.htm
Centers for Disease Control: Chemical/Biological/Radiological Hotline
   for obtaining information
   Hotline: 888-246-2675
Centers for Disease Control: National Immunization Hotline
   Hotline: 800-232-2522
Infectious Diseases Society of America
   www.idsociety.org/bt/biotemplate.cfm?template=an_summary.htm
National Institutes of Health
   www.nlm.nih.gov/medlineplus/anthrax.html
National Response Center: Chemical/Biological/Radiological Hotline
   for reporting incidents
   Hotline: 800-424-8802
State public-health locator for officials, agencies, and public hotlines
   www.statepublichealth.org
The Survival Guide: What to Do in a Biological, Chemical, or
   Nuclear Emergency website
   www.911guide.com
U.S. Army Medical Research Institute of Infectious Diseases (USAMRIID)
   www.usamriid.army.mil
   Response Line: 888-USA-RIID (888-872-7443)
   Questions or Comments: USAMRIIDweb@amedd.army.mil
U.S. Department of Defense: Vaccine immunization program
   Phone (Toll-free): 877-GET-VACC (877-438-8222)
   www.anthrax.osd.mil

BOTULISM

DISEASE	
Botulism	

ORGANISM RESPONSIBLE	TYPE
Clostridium botulinum	Toxin made by bacteria

HOW YOU GET EXPOSED

Ingestion, inhalation, or by contamination of an open wound by the live bacteria

TIME FROM EXPOSURE TO ILLNESS

FROM FOOD and INHALED: 12–72 hours

MAJOR SYMPTOMS

Increasing muscle weakness beginning in the face (blurred vision, difficulty speaking and swallowing) and progressing down the body symmetrically (left and right sides evenly) to include all muscle groups; the end stage is paralysis and respiratory failure

EMERGENCY RESPONSE

- If possible airborne release has occurred, cover nose and mouth with a wet fabric of some kind or a respiratory mask; take shallow breaths if you must breathe before out of the area
- Stay away from exposure area
- If exposed to airborne attack, wash skin, clothing, and exposed objects with soap and water
- If you are coming down with symptoms, go to a hospital (do not drive yourself)
- If available, antitoxin treatment should begin as soon as possible

TREATMENT

Antitoxin, but supplies are limited

POSSIBILITY OF DEATH

FOODBORNE: 7.5%, INHALED: Unknown, but presumably much higher than foodborne

VACCINE

Under development

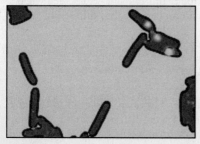

Clostridium botulinum are rod-shaped bacteria. They cause disease via the ingestion or inhalation of toxins that they produce.

WHAT IT IS

Botulism is a rare disease caused by deadly toxins made from the bacteria *Clostridium botulinum* and is usually acquired from food such as home-canned goods or fish products. It is found worldwide in soil and sometimes in animal droppings. The three main types of naturally occurring human botulism are FOODBORNE, WOUND, and INFANT BOTULISM. There are usually around 100 cases reported each year in the United States (25% foodborne, 72% infantile, 3% wound). A fourth, manmade type—INHALED BOTULISM—is the form that would most likely be used in a bioterror attack.

Botulinum bacteria go into a "spore" or resting phase when they are not getting enough nutrients from the environment and form hardy, protective shells around themselves. The bacteria themselves are usually harmless; it is when they are growing and produce harmful chemicals called toxins that they do their damage. Botulinum toxin is one of the most poisonous substances known to man; theoretically, a single gram of crystalline toxin, evenly dispersed and inhaled, would kill more than a million people.

Ironically, the botulism toxin is also used in healthcare (called MEDICINAL BOTULISM). It is used in the treatment of migraine, back pain, stroke, cerebral palsy, and cosmetically for wrinkles under the trade name Botox (a vial of therapeutic toxin contains only 0.005% of the estimated human fatal dose).

WHAT IT DOES

The toxin blocks nerve-to-muscle communication, causing the muscle to be unable to receive the nerve's message to move (paralysis). The paralysis travels down the body, eventually affecting every muscle, including those muscles that enable breathing.

HOW YOU GET EXPOSED

Botulism is not contagious. You can get exposed to the toxin by eating food contaminated with it or by breathing it in. Infant botulism is thought to result from ingested organisms producing toxin in the gut rather than from ingesting toxin-contaminated food. You can also get exposed when a wound is contaminated by the botulinum bacteria, but this is very rare.

ASSESSMENT OF RISK

Centers for Disease Control Rating = High Priority (Category A)

Risk of Use in an Attack

Botulinum bacteria is highly available. However, while all botulinum strains produce toxin, some are more deadly than others, and obtaining one of the strains that produce a deadly toxin would be difficult. It would also require sophisticated technological skills to engineer the toxin into a weaponized air spray.

Mixing the toxin into food that is normally eaten uncooked is a potential means of exposure, although foodborne botulism is not as deadly as the inhaled variety. Municipal water supplies are considered relatively safe because the toxin would not endure water-treatment processes such as chlorination; moreover, the amount necessary to successfully contaminate a reservoir would be enormous. As of 2001, no waterborne botulism has ever been reported. However, unlike treated water, the botulinum toxin can remain stable for several days in untreated water or beverages.

Some countries, such as Iran, North Korea, and Syria, are known to have experimented with the use of botulinum toxin in weapons. In the Gulf War, Iraq loaded it into bombs it deployed; its effects have not been determined.

How Dangerous Is It?

The death rate for botulism caused by contaminated food is 7.5%. The percentage could be much higher if the toxin were weaponized as a concentrated air spray and inhaled.

One of the greatest dangers is thought to be that intensive care units could become quickly overwhelmed with patients who needed breathing support in the event of a mass outbreak.

TIMELINE OF ILLNESS

FOODBORNE: Symptoms begin 2 hours to 8 days (most commonly 12–72 hours) after ingestion of contaminated food or liquid.
INHALED: Symptoms would probably begin 12–72 hours after breathing it in.

Recovery takes several months because it requires the growth of new nerve endings; full recovery could take up to a year.

SYMPTOMS

The muscle-weakening effects of botulinum toxin always begin at the head, causing blurred vision, double vision, drooping eyelids, and/or difficulty speaking and swallowing. If untreated, the paralysis will travel symmetrically down the body (rapidity and severity depend on the rate and amount of toxin absorption), affecting arms, torso, legs, and respiratory muscles. Other symptoms include generalized weakness, dry mouth, constipation, inability to urinate, dilation (enlargement) of pupils, sensitivity to light, dizziness, upset stomach, and vomiting. Because the "blood-brain barrier" keeps large molecules, including botulinum toxin, from entering the brain, the patient would be fully conscious and thinking would be unimpaired.

FOODBORNE: Above symptoms may begin with stomach cramps, nausea, vomiting, or diarrhea.

EMERGENCY RESPONSE

- **If you are in the vicinity of an expected airborne botulism attack:**
  - Cover your nose and mouth with fabric (wet if possible).
- **If you have been sprayed with airborne toxin:**
  - Wash skin, clothing, and exposed objects thoroughly with soap.
  - You can also wash with bleach solution (1 part bleach, 9 parts water) as an extra precaution. Bleach should never be used on the eyes.
  - Use a protective respiratory mask to prevent inhalation of the toxin (entry is not through intact skin).
- **If you are coming down with symptoms:**
  - Go to the hospital immediately.
  - The sooner treatment begins, the less nerve damage will occur.
  - In cases of mass exposure, unless paralysis is clearly improving, treatment (by medical professionals) should not wait for laboratory confirmation.
  - Make a travel and activity log of your previous 3 days.
  - Have someone drive you to a medical care facility; do not drive yourself.
- **If a foodborne outbreak is suspected:**
  - Cooking food at 185°F for 5 minutes will destroy the toxin.

TESTING AND DIAGNOSIS

Ruling Out Botulism and Other Considerations in Diagnosis

- Botulism does not cause fever. If you have a fever, it is probably something else.
- The way to tell the difference between a person having a stroke and a person with botulism is that in the case of stroke, paralysis will generally occur on one part or side of the body. With botulism, paralysis occurs on both left and right sides evenly as it travels from the head on down the body.
- Botulinum toxin in solution is colorless, odorless, and, as far as is known, tasteless.
- While botulinum outbreaks can occur naturally, a large outbreak caused by one of the rarer strains of the toxin would suggest a bioterrorist attack, as would the absence of a common food source of people falling ill.

Testing

- Diagnostic testing for botulism is time-consuming. When botulism is highly suspected and there is a known bioterrorist attack, treatment in patients with neurologic symptoms should begin before diagnosis is confirmed in the lab, as time is of the essence.

- Definitive laboratory tests are available at the CDC and at some state and local facilities. Contaminated food can be sampled and tested, as can blood, stool, vomit, and material from wounds. Food suspected of being contaminated should be refrigerated until retrieved for testing by public-health personnel. The Food and Drug Administration (FDA) and the U.S. Department of Agriculture (USDA) can also test food.
- Physicians may need to rule out other illnesses by performing a spinal tap, which involves injecting a needle into the spine to extract fluid. In the event of a mass attack, it would be evident to healthcare professionals that botulinum was released and additional tests such as these would not be necessary for each diagnosis.

TREATMENT

An **antitoxin** made from horse blood products blocks the toxin from circulating in the blood (though it does not reverse the paralysis that has already occurred). The "trivalent antitoxin" made for the botulinum toxin covers the 3 most common varieties that exist (A, B, and E out of types A–F). It is available only through the Centers for Disease Control and Protection (CDC). The CDC can ship it out to hospitals and doctors immediately, 24 hours a day. A "heptavalent antitoxin" also exists, which covers all 7 of the botulinum strains and is used by the U.S. Army, but it is still considered experimental.

Activated charcoal tablets may inactivate type A botulinum toxin (the type commonly found in food), though studies are inconclusive.

Intravenous (IV) fluids and nutritional support may be required.

In serious cases, if breathing muscles became paralyzed, **breathing support** such as a ventilator (breathing machine) could be required.

If an infection also occurs, aminoglycoside and tetracycline antibiotics should be avoided, as they could worsen the effects of the toxin.

VACCINE

While a vaccine that protects against types A–E has been in use for 30 years in environments considered hazardous (e.g., laboratories), it is still considered experimental. Mass immunization is neither feasible nor desirable due to side effects, scarcity of the vaccine, rarity of the natural disease, and elimination of potential benefits of medicinal botulinum toxin (see *WHAT IT IS* above).

CHILDREN

No special precautions.

PREGNANCY

Based on limited information, there is no indication that treatment of pregnant women with botulism should differ from standard therapy. The risks to fetuses of exposure to the antitoxin are unknown.

ENVIRONMENTAL DECONTAMINATION AND CLEANUP

- Environmental surfaces should be cleaned and decontaminated with a mild bleach solution (1 part household bleach, 9 parts water) in the event of an airborne exposure.
- The toxin is destroyed by boiling for 5–10 minutes.
- Substantial inactivation of the toxin occurs after about 2 days from the time of release into the air. Decontamination should not be necessary after this point.

HOW YOU CAN PREPARE

Keep activated charcoal on hand.

Keep health-facility and emergency phone numbers readily available (see *ADDITIONAL RESOURCES* below and the *Public Resources and Contact Information* section of the book).

ADDITIONAL RESOURCES

American College of Physicians–American Society of Internal Medicine
    www.acponline.org/bioterro/biotoxin.htm
Centers for Disease Control (CDC)
    www.bt.cdc.gov/agent/botulism/index.asp
    www.cdc.gov/ncidod/dbmd/diseaseinfo/botulism_g.htm
Centers for Disease Control: Chemical/Biological/Radiological Hotline
    for obtaining information Hotline: 888-246-2675
Centers for Disease Control: National Immunization Hotline
    Hotline: 800-232-2522
Food and Drug Administration (FDA) website: *www.fda.gov*
National Institutes of Health
    www.nlm.nih.gov/medlineplus/botulism.html
    www.nlm.nih.gov/medlineplus/ency/article/001384.htm
National Response Center: Chemical/Biological/Radiological Hotline
    for reporting incidents Hotline: 800-424-8802
State public-health locator for officials, agencies, and public hotlines
    www.statepublichealth.org
U.S. Department of Agriculture (USDA)
    www.usda.gov

BRUCELLOSIS

DISEASE
Brucellosis

ORGANISM RESPONSIBLE	TYPE
Brucellae	Bacteria

HOW YOU CATCH IT

Ingestion of or contact with contaminated animals or animal products, or by inhalation; person-to-person transmission possible but unlikely

TIME FROM EXPOSURE TO ILLNESS

2–3 weeks

MAJOR SYMPTOMS

Flulike symptoms such as fever, chills, sweats, headache, joint or back pain, loss of appetite, cough, chest pain made worse by breathing; chronic form could cause mental status changes such as anxiety and depression

EMERGENCY RESPONSE

- If possible airborne release has occurred, cover your mouth and nose with fabric (wet if possible) or an N95 respiratory mask
- Wash potentially contaminated body parts immediately with soap and water
- Begin antibiotic treatment as soon as possible if high suspicion of infection

TREATMENT

Two antibiotics: doxycycline and either gentamicin, streptomycin, or rifampin

POSSIBILITY OF DEATH

2–5%

VACCINE

None available

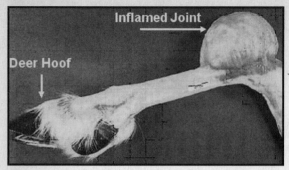

Infection and inflammation involving the knee joint of a caribou with brucellosis. Humans with brucellosis may experience joint pain and arthritis but inflammation would not reach this degree of swelling.

WHAT IT IS

Brucellosis is an infectious, multisystem disease caused by one of six kinds of bacteria of the genus *Brucella* and is usually passed among animals (e.g., sheep, goats, cattle, deer, elk, pigs, dogs). It occurs worldwide but is not very common in the United States. Of the 100–200 human cases in the United States per year, the majority are related to the farm animal industry or occur in laboratory workers who studied the bacteria.

WHAT IT DOES

When *Brucella* bacteria get inside humans and animals, they travel to the lymphatic system (part of the immune system), where they replicate within lymph nodes. From there they enter the bloodstream and spread throughout the body. Abscesses can form in tissues and organs, such as in lymph tissue, the liver, the spleen, and in bone marrow.

Brucellae enter certain cells of the immune system (white blood cells) that are designed to rid the body of harmful substances, thus dodging their destructive effects. Once the bacteria are inside these cells, an envelope forms around them for protection. Within this shell, the bacteria grow and reproduce, eventually breaking out and killing the host cell, at which point they are released into the bloodstream. This cycle explains why fevers and other symptoms come and go: symptoms recur whenever there is a new release of bacteria into the bloodstream.

HOW YOU CATCH IT

Humans usually become infected by coming into contact with animals or animal products that are contaminated with *Brucella* organisms, such as by ingestion or through an open skin wound. The most common way to contract brucellosis is by eating or drinking contaminated milk products. It could also be contracted by inhaling infectious aerosols.

Extremely rare cases have been reported of infant infection through mother's breast milk and of sexual transmission. Once an infected person begins treatment, he would probably not be infectious after 3 days.

ASSESSMENT OF RISK

Centers for Disease Control Rating = Second-Highest Priority (Category B)

Risk of Use in an Attack
Of the four types of brucellae that can infect humans, the two species that are most considered potential biological terrorism agents are *Brucella melitensis* and *Brucella suis.* Aspects that might make it attractive to terrorists are:
1) It could be highly infectious if delivered by air.
2) It is fairly stable in the environment, as it survives for 6 weeks in dust and 10 weeks in soil or water.
3) It is found in the environment.
4) Its lingering effects would prolong the attack for many people.

How Dangerous Is It?
Many infected with brucellae in natural epidemics never come down with symptoms. However, it would be highly infectious via the aerosol route: if only 10–100 bacteria were inhaled by a person, it could cause disease.

Deaths caused by brucellosis would be rare. The 2–5% of fatal cases are usually caused from spread of the infection to the heart or brain.

TIMELINE OF ILLNESS

Time from exposure to illness is relatively long (usually 2–3 weeks) but can be highly variable (5–60 days). Large airborne doses could shorten the time to illness and increase the clinical symptoms.

Relapses are common; recovery would be prolonged, even with antibiotic therapy. Without treatment, it could become a lifelong, chronic disease.

SYMPTOMS

Symptoms are extremely variable from person to person. Initially, flulike symptoms usually occur, such as fever, chills, sweats, headache, joint or back pain, loss of appetite, cough, and/or chest pain made worse by breathing. Gastrointestinal symptoms occur in up to 70% of cases (less so in children), such as nausea, vomiting, abdominal pain, and diarrhea or constipation. Less than 5% of sufferers will exhibit a skin rash of pus-filled blisters.

Brucellosis can also cause long-lasting or chronic symptoms ranging from 2–12 months, including fever, arthritis, and swollen testicles in males.

With proper treatment, symptoms beyond 12 months are rare but possible and would primarily involve recurrent fever, malaise, bone or joint pain/arthritis, headache, chronic fatigue, anxiety, and depression.

EMERGENCY RESPONSE

- **If possible airborne release has occurred,** cover your mouth and nose with fabric (wet if possible) or an N95 respiratory mask.

- **If potentially contaminated by airborne *Brucella* bacteria, wash** hands and body with antimicrobial soap. Bodily sites exposed to blood, body fluids, secretions, or excretions from patients with suspected brucellosis infections should be immediately washed with soap and water.

- **Brucellae can be rapidly killed with disinfectants.** Objects and surfaces in the immediate area of an airborne release may be cleaned with a 0.5% bleach solution (1 part household bleach added to 9 parts water). Listen to instructions from emergency management personnel.

- **Begin antibiotic treatment** as soon as possible if infection is strongly suspected.

- **Wear a protective N95 respiratory mask** around infected patients.

TESTING AND DIAGNOSIS

Brucellosis is so rarely contracted in humans in the United States that many physicians might not do the proper testing and miss the diagnosis.

Brucellosis is definitively diagnosed in a laboratory by finding *Brucella* organisms in samples of blood or bone marrow (called a positive culture). Blood tests can also be performed that detect antibodies against the bacteria; if this method is used, 2 blood samples should be collected 2 weeks apart. It should be noted that due to the nature of the tests, there is a moderate degree of false results.

A promising new test involves DNA testing (extracted from a blood sample). For a DNA polymerase chain reaction test, the results are available in about an hour.

TREATMENT

Begin **antibiotic therapy** as soon as possible if contaminated with weaponized brucellae. Two different antibiotics at the same time are recommended due to the high relapse rate that occurs with single-drug treatment. Doxycycline is advised for 6 weeks, along with either a gentamicin, streptomycin, or rifampin regimen for 7–10 days (note that high-fat meals will interfere with the absorption of rifampin).

Dehydrated patients should receive **dextrose** (sugar) and **electrolyte solutions** by IV if possible.

If breathing becomes compromised, a **breathing tube** or **ventilator** (breathing machine) may be necessary.

If, despite adequate therapy, fever or symptoms persist, an examination should be performed to **search for abscesses that may need to be drained.**

For NEUROBRUCELLOSIS, the recommended antibiotic combination is gentamicin plus either doxycycline or trimethoprim-sulfamethoxazole (TMP/SMX, sold under the brand name Bactrim), *plus* rifampin. This regimen should last for a minimum of 8 weeks.

VACCINE

None commercially available.

CHILDREN

– For children over 8 years of age with uncomplicated brucellosis, the recommended treatment is: doxycycline *plus* gentamicin, streptomycin, or rifampin for the same length of time as the adult recommendation. For children less than 8 years: trimethoprim-sulfamethoxazole (TMP/SMX) *plus* gentamicin.

PREGNANCY

– Pregnant women should substitute doxycycline with the 2–antibiotic drug, trimethoprim-sulfamethoxazole (TMP/SMX), *plus* rifampin.

SPECIAL PRECAUTIONS

The sooner antibiotic treatment can be initiated, the better the chances are that chronic, lifelong brucellosis will be avoided.

ENVIRONMENTAL DECONTAMINATION AND CLEANUP

– Left alone, *Brucella* bacteria may survive for 6 weeks in dust and up to 10 weeks in soil or water, but they are easily killed with disinfectants.

– Decontamination can be accomplished with a 0.5% sodium hypochlorite solution (1 part household bleach added to 9 parts water).

– The bacteria are killed at 145°F for 30 minutes. Thus, thoroughly cooking food would prevent brucellosis by ingestion.

– Routine washing of clothing would destroy the bacteria on fabric.

- Proper treatment of water, through boiling, chlorination, or iodination would be important in areas intentionally subjected to brucellae aerosols.

HOW YOU CAN PREPARE

Wash hands regularly. As the majority of all infections are spread this way, adopting this habit will prevent everyday infections as well.

Keep an N95 respiratory mask on hand.

Keep health-facility and emergency phone numbers readily available (see *ADDITIONAL RESOURCES* below and the *Public Resources and Contact Information* section of the book). In the event of an attack, antibiotic treatment should begin immediately.

On self-prescribing antibiotics: Unnecessary and frequent use of antibiotics could kill the weakest bacteria and leave the strongest to keep reproducing and infecting others. In this way, we could build antibiotic-resistant bacteria, or bacteria that cannot be killed by common (or possibly any) antibiotics. Furthermore, allergic reactions to antibiotics are not uncommon and can even be life-threatening, and they may also cross-react with other medications you are taking.

ADDITIONAL RESOURCES

Centers for Disease Control (CDC)
  www.bt.cdc.gov/agent/brucellosis/index.asp
Centers for Disease Control: Chemical/Biological/Radiological Hotline
  for obtaining information
  Hotline: 888-246-2675
National Institutes of Health: Medical encyclopedia
  www.nlm.nih.gov/medlineplus/ency/article/000597.htm
National Response Center: Chemical/Biological/Radiological Hotline
  for reporting incidents
  Hotline: 800-424-8802
State public-health locator for officials, agencies, and public hotlines
  www.statepublichealth.org
The Survival Guide: What to Do in a Biological, Chemical, or Nuclear
  Emergency website: For updates, supplementary information, and
  helpful links
  www.911guide.com

GLANDERS

DISEASE	
Glanders	

ORGANISM RESPONSIBLE	TYPE
Burkholderia mallei	Bacteria

HOW YOU CATCH IT

Bacteria get into the body through mucous membranes (such as mouth, eyes, or lining of the nose), an opening in the skin like a scratch or cut, or by breathing them in; in nature the disease is usually passed to humans from horses, donkeys, or mules

TIME FROM EXPOSURE TO ILLNESS

THROUGH SKIN OR MUCOUS MEMBRANES: 1–5 days
INHALED (form most likely to be used in an attack): 10–14 days

MAJOR SYMPTOMS

THROUGH SKIN OR MEMBRANES: Ulcer formation on the skin at site of bacterial entry, swollen lymph nodes, mucus production from the nose and mouth
INHALED: High fever, chills, sweats, body aches, headache, swollen neck glands, chest pain, congestion, pneumonia; open sores on mucous membranes and internal organs; a dark pink, pus-filled rash can also develop

EMERGENCY RESPONSE

– If possible airborne release has occurred, cover nose and mouth with fabric (wet if possible) or an N95 respiratory mask and leave the immediate vicinity
– If you think you might have been exposed, wash skin thoroughly with soap and water
– Hold eyes under running water for 15 minutes
– If there is an attack in your area and you develop a fever, call your doctor

TREATMENT

Antibiotics such as amoxicillin and clavulanate combined, Bactrim, ceftazidime, or tetracycline, among many others, for 60–150 days

POSSIBILITY OF DEATH

Death rate of 100% within 1 month would be expected without antibiotics; rapid initiation of antibiotic treatment should decrease this, but there is little data available

VACCINE

None

WHAT IT IS

Glanders, a potentially deadly disease caused by the bacteria *Burkholderia mallei*, is most often found in animals like horses, donkeys, and mules, but humans can get it, too. There are four main forms, and which kind you get depends on how you contract it: the SKIN AND MUSCLE (or SOFT-TISSUE) FORM is usually caused from acquiring the bacteria through a break in the skin or through mucous membranes; the LUNG FORM is caught by breathing it in and results in flulike symptoms and extreme lung congestion; the BLOODSTREAM INFECTION results when bacteria multiply and circulate throughout the bloodstream and can be rapidly fatal; and the CHRONIC FORM, which is generally acquired through the skin and can persist for years, causes multiple abscesses on the skin and muscles of the arms and legs and is also associated with enlarging and hardening of the lymph nodes near the site of infection.

The symptoms and treatment of glanders are very similar to melioidosis, though the natural habitat and mode of infection of the bacteria are different (see Chapter 5). Glanders is commonly seen among domestic animals in Africa, Asia, the Middle East, and Central and South America. Other than among laboratory employees who worked with the *Burkholderia mallei* bacteria, there have been no naturally occurring cases of glanders in the United States in over 60 years. Hence, an outbreak of this disease in the United States would very likely be due to a deliberate attack.

WHAT IT DOES

The LUNG or INHALED FORM is the type most likely to be used in a bioterrorist attack. If the glanders bacteria were made into a weapon to be sprayed into the air and breathed in, the bacteria would get into the body through the lungs and multiply, causing a pneumonia-like infection. It could then spread throughout the body, infecting many organs. Whatever part of the body it infects, it often causes ulcers—like canker sores—even in many organs, including the lungs. If mucous membranes become infected, bleeding ulcers will form there, and if skin becomes infected, pus-filled bumps will develop. If it spreads throughout the bloodstream, it is usually fatal.

HOW YOU CATCH IT

The bacteria can get into the body through mucous membranes in the mouth, eyes, or lining of the nose. It can also be acquired through an opening in the skin like a cut or abrasion. In nature, you can only catch the disease from a live animal, as the bacteria that cause glanders do not grow in water, soil, or plants. The bacteria can also cause infection by inhalation.

Person-to-person transmission would be highly unlikely, though not impossible. It could occur through direct contact with infected sores or the discharge from the sores of a glanders patient.

ASSESSMENT OF RISK

Centers for Disease Control Rating = Second-Highest Priority (Category B)

Risk of Use in an Attack

Though most people have never heard of glanders, it has been studied by nations with bioweapons programs since at least World War I. It is considered to be a possible choice of use in an attack because of its deadliness without antibiotic treatment, the extended treatment period required, its ability to cause illness for years to come, and the small amount needed to launch the disease.

How Dangerous Is It?

It does not take many bacteria to produce an infection; in fact, as few as 1–10 can be lethal to an animal (and presumably a person as well). It is extremely deadly, with most patients expected to die within 1 month without antibiotics. The BLOODSTREAM form has been uniformly fatal. Even with rapid antibiotic treatment of glanders, mortality could be high, though there is not much data available since the disease had largely disappeared by the time many antibiotics became available.

TIMELINE OF ILLNESS

LOCALIZED SKIN INFECTION: An ulcer usually forms on the skin 1–5 days after exposure to the bacteria.
INHALED FORM: Symptoms (see below) would begin 10–14 days after exposure. Death could follow in 3–4 weeks if not treated with antibiotics.

SYMPTOMS

Generalized symptoms of glanders include fever, muscle aches, chest pain, muscle tightness, and headache. Additional symptoms have included excessive tearing of the eyes, light sensitivity, and diarrhea.

SKIN AND MUSCLE FORM: This form of infection is usually expressed as an ulcer on the skin at the point of bacterial entry, such as a cut or abrasion. Swollen lymph nodes may also be apparent. Infections involving the mucous membranes of the eyes, nose, and respiratory tract will cause purulent (mucus containing pus) production at the affected sites. The acute form may produce fever and general muscle aches, and it could progress rapidly to infect the bloodstream.

LUNG (INHALED) FORM: Symptoms are high fever (102°F or higher), chills, sweats, muscle aches, headache, chest pain, swollen neck glands (lymph nodes), a diffuse skin rash, sensitivity to light, jaundice (a yellow cast to the skin), and diarrhea. Other complaints are extreme congestion due to thick mucus in the lungs. Sometimes the disease causes a rash of pus-filled bumps to erupt on the skin. Bloody nodules or ulcers may form in mucous membranes—such as in nasal passages, eyes, or lips—causing blood-streaked discharge; death can follow within days.

BLOODSTREAM INFECTION: Glanders bloodstream infections carry the bacteria throughout the body. It is usually fatal within 7–10 days.

CHRONIC FORM: The primary symptoms of this form, which is generally acquired through the skin, may not present for some time. They are bumps or ulcers forming on the skin; followed by abscesses on organs, bones, and muscles, causing joint and muscle pain; and swollen lymph nodes near the site of infection. Symptoms could continue to flare up for years. An aerosolized attack would not likely produce this form.

EMERGENCY RESPONSE

- **If possible airborne release has occurred, cover nose and mouth with fabric** (wet if possible) or an N95 respiratory mask and leave the immediate vicinity.
- **If you think you might have been exposed,** wash intact skin thoroughly with soap and running water. Cut skin should be encouraged to bleed and then placed under running water.
- **If your eyes have been exposed,** run room-temperature water over them for 15 minutes.
- **If there is an attack in your area and you develop a fever,** call your doctor. Keep an especially close eye on the most vulnerable population: young children, the elderly, and people with deficient immune systems.
- **Post-exposure treatment to prevent the disease** from developing may be recommended with the drug trimethoprim-sulfamethoxazole (TMP/SMX) or other antibiotics.
- **If in the presence of a patient or suspected patient with glanders disease,** a surgical mask, face shield, and gown (or the like) should be worn.
- **Heating to 165°F** would kill the bacteria.

TESTING AND DIAGNOSIS

Glanders is very difficult to diagnose because it resembles many other diseases and there is no easy test to confirm the diagnosis. Antibody testing can assist in diagnosis, but the results are not available for over 2–3 weeks.

Microscopic staining tests are useful diagnostic tools, although they are not specific. Blood cultures are usually negative and are therefore not helpful in confirming diagnosis.

A chest x-ray would be helpful to aid in diagnosis, as it would show pneumonia as well as nodules and abscesses in the lungs.

TREATMENT

Antibiotic treatment is the best defense against glanders. Note that not all strains of *Burkholderia mallei* will be killed by the same antibiotics; only your doctor or an authorized public-health official will be able to tell you which will work best in a given outbreak. In general, the antibiotics of choice are: amoxicillin and clavulanate combined, trimethoprim-sulfamethoxazole (TMP/SMX, also known as Bactrim), tetracycline, or third-generation cephalosporins such as ceftazidime. Though experience in humans is limited, the following antibiotics have also been shown to be effective in laboratory tests: gentamicin, imipenem, doxycycline, and ciprofloxacin. Treatment period may be 60–150 days.

For the most severe cases, the U.S. Army recommends combining 2 drug treatments from above for 30 days, and then continuing with one medication for the next 5–11 months. Ceftazidime and Bactrim is the preferred combination.

As stated above, the treatment period could last up to a year. It is extremely important that the entire regimen be completed, as the disease could recur and be fatal. In addition, bacteria resistant to antibiotics could emerge if the full therapy term is not carried out.

Post-exposure treatment to prevent the disease from developing may be recommended with the drug TMP/SMX (Bactrim).

Large amounts of **intravenous (IV) fluids** may be necessary if the blood pressure drops, which usually occurs when the infection spreads to the bloodstream.

Surgical drainage of abscesses may be required.

VACCINE
There is no vaccine available at this time.

CHILDREN
- Young children are more susceptible to catching glanders than are adults.
- Though tetracycline and doxycycline are recommeneded treatments for adults, they are not recommended for children less than 8 years old. Otherwise, treatment is the same for children as for adults but with adjusted doses.

PREGNANCY

Amoxicillin-clavulanic acid and ceftazidime are usually safe but have some risks associated with pregnancy, hence the benefits to taking them must outweigh their risks. The safety of SMX/TMP (Bactrim) has not been established during pregnancy. Though tetracycline and doxycycline are recommended treatments for adults, they are not recommended for pregnant women. The use of any of these drugs during pregnancy should be discussed with your doctor.

SPECIAL PRECAUTIONS

The bacteria that cause glanders are extremely difficult to get rid of, which is why such an extensive period of antibiotic therapy is required. The symptoms, and the infection itself, can actually occur years or even *decades* later, even if the patient did not initially come down with the disease.

ENVIRONMENTAL DECONTAMINATION AND CLEANUP

- The ultraviolet rays of sunlight would kill the glanders bacteria in the course of several hours.
- Standard disinfectants and germicides, such as 0.5% hypochlorite bleach solution (1 part bleach, 9 parts water), are effective to decontaminate an area.

HOW YOU CAN PREPARE

Have on hand: a disinfectant, such as a germicide or mild bleach solution, to decontaminate surfaces, and an N95 respiratory mask.

Keep health-facility and emergency phone numbers readily available (see *ADDITIONAL RESOURCES* below and the *Public Resources and Contact Information* section of the book).

On self-prescribing antibiotics: Unnecessary and frequent use of antibiotics could lead to the production of antibiotic-resistant bacteria. In addition, allergic reactions to antibiotics are not uncommon, and they can cross-react with other medications as well.

ADDITIONAL RESOURCES

Centers for Disease Control (CDC)
   www.cdc.gov/ncidod/dbmd/diseaseinfo/glanders_g.htm
Centers for Disease Control: Chemical/Biological/Radiological Hotline
   for obtaining information: 888-246-2675
National Response Center: Chemical/Biological/Radiological Hotline
   for reporting incidents: 800-424-8802
State public-health locator for officials, agencies, and public hotlines
   www.statepublichealth.org

MELIOIDOSIS

DISEASE	
Melioidosis	

ORGANISM RESPONSIBLE	TYPE
Burkholderia pseudomallei	Bacteria

HOW YOU CATCH IT

By direct contact with contaminated soil or water (especially through skin abrasions) or by breathing in contaminated dust or water; person-to-person transmission can occur

TIME FROM EXPOSURE TO ILLNESS

Not clearly defined, could be 2 days to many years

MAJOR SYMPTOMS

ACQUIRED THROUGH SKIN: Bump forms at the point of bacterial entry on the skin; acute form may produce fever and general muscle aches and could progress rapidly to infect the bloodstream

INHALED (most likely form in bioterror attack): High fever, chills, sweats, body aches, headache, swollen glands in the neck, chest pain, cough, congestion, pneumonia; could also lead to open sores on mucous membranes and internal organs as well as a dark pink, pus-filled rash

EMERGENCY RESPONSE

- If possible airborne release has occurred, cover nose and mouth with fabric (wet if possible) or an N95 respiratory mask and leave the immediate vicinity
- If you think you might have been exposed, wash skin thoroughly with soap and water
- Hold eyes under running water for 15 minutes
- If there is an attack in your area and you develop a fever, call your doctor

TREATMENT

Antibiotics such as amoxicillin and clavulanate combined, TMX/SMP (Bactrim), ceftazidime, or tetracycline, for 60–150 days

POSSIBILITY OF DEATH

Overall, around 30%; can be as high as 95% without treatment

VACCINE

None

WHAT IT IS

Melioidosis, also known as Whitmore's disease, is an infectious disease caused by the bacteria *Burkholderia pseudomallei*. The symptoms and treatment are very similar to those for glanders disease (though the natural habitat and mode of infection of the bacteria are different). The severity of infection could range from no illness to severe illness requiring hospitalization.

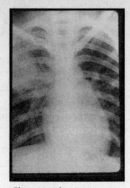

Chest x-ray showing melioidosis infection involving the right upper lung.

The bacteria that cause melioidosis are found in soil and surface water in predominantly tropical climates, especially Southeast Asia (e.g., Vietnam, Cambodia, Laos, Thailand, Malaysia, Burma). They are also found in northern Australia, the South Pacific, Africa, India, and the Middle East. About 0–5 cases are reported in the United States each year, usually occurring among travelers, immigrants, and IV drug users. In addition to humans, many different animals can be infected via contaminated soil and water—including sheep, goats, horses, pigs, cattle, dogs, cats, and rodents.

There are four main forms that can develop, which depend on how you contract it: a SKIN AND MUSCLE (or SOFT-TISSUE) FORM, which is usually acquired through a break in the skin; a LUNG FORM, which is caught by inhaling the bacteria and causes mild bronchitis to severe pneumonia; a BLOODSTREAM INFECTION, usually affecting certain vulnerable patients such as people with AIDS, and can be rapidly fatal; and finally, a CHRONIC FORM, which can come and go for years and affects the joints, lymph nodes, and possibly the skin, brain, liver, lungs, bones, and spleen.

WHAT IT DOES

SKIN AND MUSCLE FORM: A nodule forms on the skin as a result of the bacteria getting in through a break in the skin. The infection could stay localized to the site of entry, or it could spread to the bloodstream.
LUNG (INHALED) FORM: Caught in nature by inhaling contaminated dust, this form is the most likely to be used in a terrorist attack. If the melioidosis bacteria were made into a weapon to be sprayed into the air and breathed in, the bacteria would get into the body through the lungs and multiply, causing a pneumonia-like infection. From the lungs this infection can spread through the bloodstream to other parts of the body.

BLOODSTREAM INFECTION: The bacteria multiply in the bloodstream and spread the infection throughout the body. This form is fatal in 95% of untreated patients, which is decreased to 30–40% if patients are treated. About one-fourth will relapse.

CHRONIC FORM: This infection causes multiple abscesses in many internal organs of the body. It can stay dormant for years and then recur.

HOW YOU CATCH IT

In nature, transmission occurs by direct contact with contaminated soil or water (especially through skin abrasions) or by breathing in contaminated dust or water. If the bacteria were weaponized into an airborne spray, you would catch the infection by breathing the bacteria into your lungs.

Person-to-person transmission is possible; it has been documented in family members who had close contact with infected household members, and 2 cases of sexual transmission have been reported.

ASSESSMENT OF RISK

Centers for Disease Control Rating = Second-Highest Priority (Category B)

Risk of Use in an Attack

Burkholderia pseudomallei has been studied by nations with bioweapons programs; it was studied by the United States for potential use but was never weaponized. It is considered to be a possible choice of use in an attack because of its deadliness without antibiotic treatment, the extended treatment period required, the ability for the bacteria to cause illness for many years, and the small amount of bacteria needed to produce the disease. It is very similar to the bacteria that cause glanders but has the advantage of being able to survive in the environment after its release.

How Dangerous Is It?

It is presumed that it would not take many bacteria to cause infection. However, though melioidosis was once considered a deadly disease (untreated, the possibility of death can be as high as 95%), the outlook for patients is now improved with proper antibiotic treatment. Treated, the possibility of death is estimated to be around 20%. One exception to this is a bloodstream infection with melioidosis, as even with appropriate therapy it could be fatal in 30–40% of patients.

TIMELINE OF ILLNESS

SKIN AND MUSCLE FORM: Time from exposure to illness is about 1–5 days.

LUNG FORM: Time from exposure to illness is about 10–14 days. Death could follow in 3–4 weeks if not treated with antibiotics.

BLOODSTREAM INFECTION: When melioidosis bacteria are dispersed throughout the body via the bloodstream, it is usually fatal within 24–48 hours without treatment.

CHRONIC FORM: A patient with chronic melioidosis can remain without symptoms for prolonged periods and reactivate years after the initial infection.

SYMPTOMS

In some cases the illness may appear more slowly, with symptoms of weight loss, intermittent fever, chest or abdominal pain, and a cough. Some people may develop skin ulcers (like canker sores) or abscesses or boils on the skin, bones, liver, spleen, or other internal organs. It is important to note that a melioidosis skin infection or ulcer on mucous membranes (e.g., in nasal passages, eyes, or mouth) should not be taken lightly, as the bacteria could get into the bloodstream and spread throughout the body.

SKIN AND MUSCLE FORM: This form of infection is usually expressed as a nodule on the skin at the point of bacterial entry, such as a break in the skin. The acute form may produce fever and general muscle aches, and it could progress rapidly to infect the bloodstream.

LUNG FORM: This form of the disease can cause anywhere from mild bronchitis to severe pneumonia. Primary symptoms are high fever (102°F or higher), chills, sweats, muscle soreness, dry cough, headache, chest pain, swollen neck glands (lymph nodes), and loss of appetite. It can progress to a bloodstream infection.

BLOODSTREAM INFECTION: Symptoms generally include breathing difficulties (respiratory distress), severe headache, fever, diarrhea, development of pus-filled bumps on the skin, muscle tenderness, and disorientation. Abscesses will be found throughout the body. It can be fatal within 24–48 hours.

CHRONIC FORM: Primary symptoms would be bumps or ulcers forming on the skin at the point of bacterial entry (e.g., a break in the skin), joint and muscle pain (due to ulcers developing on muscles), and swollen lymph nodes. Abscesses could form on the brain, liver, lungs, bones, and spleen. Symptoms could continue to flare up for years, usually triggered by debilitating factors such as major surgery, extensive burns, or malnutrition.

EMERGENCY RESPONSE

- **If possible airborne release has occurred, cover nose and mouth with fabric** (wet if possible) or an N95 respiratory mask and leave the immediate vicinity.

- **If you think you might have been exposed to the melioidosis bacteria,** wash intact skin thoroughly with soap and running water. Cut skin should be encouraged to bleed and then placed under running water.

- **If your eyes have been exposed**, run room-temperature water over them for 15 minutes.

- **If there is an attack in your area and you develop a fever**, call your doctor. Keep an especially close eye on those most vulnerable: young children, the elderly, and people with deficient immune systems.

- **If in the presence of a patient or suspected patient with melioidosis**, contact and respiratory precautions should be taken, such as wearing a surgical mask, face shield, gown, and gloves.

- **Heating to 165°F** would kill the bacteria.

TESTING AND DIAGNOSIS

Melioidosis cannot be diagnosed by clinical symptoms alone because it resembles many other diseases. Antibody testing can assist in diagnosis but the results take a long time. Microscopic staining tests are useful diagnostic tools, although they are not specific, either. Blood, phlegm, skin lesion, and urine cultures are helpful in making a diagnosis.

A chest x-ray would be a helpful aid in diagnosis, as it would show pneumonia as well as nodules and abscesses in the lungs. However, the x-ray pattern could be confused with that of tuberculosis or other lung conditions.

TREATMENT

Antibiotic treatment is the best defense against melioidosis. In general, the antibiotics of choice are: amoxicillin and clavulanate combined, trimethoprim-sulfamethoxazole (TMP/SMX, also known as Bactrim), or tetracycline for 60–150 days. Though experience in humans is limited, ceftazidime and other antibiotics have also been effective in laboratory tests.

For the most severe cases, the U.S. Army recommends combining 2 drug treatments mentioned above for 30 days, and then continuing with one medication for the next 5–11 months. Ceftazidime and Bactrim are the preferred combination.

As stated above, the treatment period could last up to a year. It is extremely important that the entire regimen be completed, as the disease could recur and be fatal. In addition, bacteria resistant to antibiotics could emerge if the full therapy term is not carried out.

Post-exposure treatment to prevent the disease from developing could be attempted with the drug TMP/SMX (Bactrim), but there is no proof this is effective.

Large amounts of **intravenous (IV) fluids** may be necessary for patients with bloodstream infection.

Surgical drainage of the abscesses may be required.

VACCINE

There is no vaccine available at this time.

CHILDREN

– Young children are more susceptible to catching melioidosis than are adults.
– Though tetracycline is one of the recommended treatments for adults, it is not recommended for children less than 8 years old. TMP/SMX is not recommended for very young children. Otherwise, treatment is the same for children as for adults but with adjusted doses.

PREGNANCY

– Amoxicillin-clavulanic acid and ceftazidime are usually safe but have some risks associated with pregnancy, hence the benefits to taking them must outweigh their risks. The safety of SMX/TMP (Bactrim) has not been established during pregnancy. Though tetracycline is one of the recommended treatments for adults, it is not recommended for pregnant women. The use of any of these drugs during pregnancy should be discussed with your doctor.

SPECIAL PRECAUTIONS

If you have any of the following conditions, you are at particular risk for contracting melioidosis if exposed to the bacteria: diabetes, chronic heavy alcohol consumption, kidney disease, lung disease, cancer, receiving steroid therapy, AIDS, and/or cuts or sores in your skin.

The bacteria that cause melioidosis are extremely difficult to get rid of, which is why such an extensive period of antibiotic therapy is required. The symptoms, and the infection itself, can actually recur years or even *decades* later.

ENVIRONMENTAL DECONTAMINATION AND CLEANUP

- The ultraviolet rays of sunlight would kill the melioidosis bacteria in the course of several hours.
- Decontamination of surfaces can be accomplished with standard disinfectants and germicides, such as a 0.5% sodium hypochlorite solution (1 part household bleach added to 9 parts water).

HOW YOU CAN PREPARE

Have on hand: a disinfectant, such as a germicide or mild bleach solution, to decontaminate nonliving surfaces, and an N95 respiratory mask.

Keep health-facility and emergency phone numbers readily available (see *ADDITIONAL RESOURCES* below and the *Public Resources and Contact Information*, section of the book).

On self-prescribing antibiotics: Unnecessary and frequent use of antibiotics could kill the weakest bacteria and leave the strongest to keep reproducing and infecting others. In this way, we could build antibiotic-resistant bacteria, or bacteria that cannot be killed by common (or possibly any) antibiotics. Furthermore, allergic reactions to antibiotics are not uncommon and can even be life-threatening, and they may also cross-react with other medications you are taking.

ADDITIONAL RESOURCES

Centers for Disease Control (CDC)
    www.cdc.gov/ncidod/dbmd/diseaseinfo/melioidosis_g.htm
Centers for Disease Control: Chemical/Biological/Radiological Hotline
    for obtaining information
    Hotline: 888-246-2675
National Response Center: Chemical/Biological/Radiological Hotline
    for reporting incidents
    Hotline: 800-424-8802
New York City Department of Health
    www.nyc.gov/html/doh/html/cd/cdmel.html
State public-health locator for officials, agencies, and public hotlines
    www.statepublichealth.org
The Survival Guide: What to Do in a Biological, Chemical, or Nuclear
    Emergency website: For updates, supplementary information, and
    helpful links
    www.911guide.com

U.S. Army Medical Research Institute of Infectious Diseases (USAMRIID)
www.usamriid.army.mil
Response Line: 888-USA-RIID (888-872-7443)
Questions or Comments: USAMRIIDweb@amedd.army.mil

PLAGUE

DISEASE

Bubonic Plague, Pneumonic Plague, and Septicemic Plague

ORGANISM RESPONSIBLE	TYPE
Yersinia pestis	Bacteria

HOW YOU CATCH IT

Breathing in bacteria, bites from infected fleas, contact with open skin infected with bacteria

TIME FROM EXPOSURE TO ILLNESS

1–8 days

MAJOR SYMPTOMS

Early symptoms can include fever, upset stomach, vomiting, diarrhea, and muscle aches
BUBONIC: High fever; swollen, tender lymph nodes (most often in the groin area)
PNEUMONIC (most likely form in bioterror attack): Fever 2–4 days after exposure; then severe pneumonia-like symptoms with cough, chest pain, coughing up blood
SEPTICEMIC: Severe fever, no swollen lymph nodes, rapid progression to multiple organ failure

EMERGENCY RESPONSE

- Stay away from outbreak area
- Use an N95 respiratory mask to avoid inhaling the bacteria; if not available cover nose and mouth with cloth (wet if possible)
- If exposed to infected person or airborne release, wash thoroughly, including eyes and mucous membranes
- Begin antibiotic treatment immediately if potentially exposed
- Decontaminate exposed materials such as clothing and bedding

TREATMENT

Antibiotics such as doxycycline, tetracycline, streptomycin, and gentamicin

POSSIBILITY OF DEATH

If untreated,
BUBONIC: 50–60%   PNEUMONIC: Up to 100%   SEPTICEMIC: Up to 100%

VACCINE

Vaccine was discontinued; new one in development

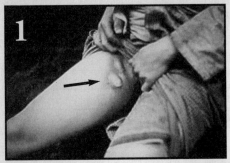

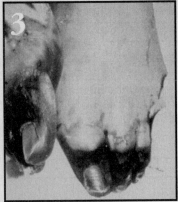

1) Enlarged femoral lymph nodes; this is the most common site of tender, swollen nodes in bubonic plague patients.

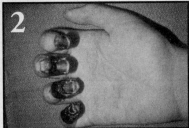

2–3) Tissue death (acral necrosis) of the fingers and toes of a person with plague.

WHAT IT IS

Plague is a disease caused by the bacteria *Yersinia pestis.* It is ordinarily found in animals, particularly rats and other rodents, birds, and pigs, and it can be found in every populated continent except Australia. There are about 1,700 cases reported annually worldwide (including 5–15 in the western United States).

There are three main types of plague—BUBONIC, PNEUMONIC, and SEPTICEMIC—all caused by the same microorganism. The way the disease is manifested usually depends upon how the bacteria enter the body.

Throughout history, plague has caused millions of deaths worldwide. The great plagues of the past have been bubonic, passed to humans by the bite of a flea that has fed on an infected rodent. In Europe in the fourteenth century, bubonic plague, called the "black death," killed 25 million people—approximately one quarter of the population. A bioterrorist attack in modern times would probably involve aerosolized *Yersinia pestis*, which would result in pneumonic plague.

WHAT IT DOES

BUBONIC	The bacteria multiply in the lymph nodes—most often in the groin and armpits—characteristically causing swelling there. Once they multiply in the lymphatic system (which normally helps rid the body of foreign invaders like viruses and bacteria), they can then spread to the lungs and bloodstream.
PNEUMONIC	The bacteria travel to the lungs and launch an infection there, causing life-threatening pneumonia.
SEPTICEMIC	Bacteria of the initial infection bypass the lymphatic system and multiply in the bloodstream, infecting and damaging all internal organs and causing blood vessels to rupture and bleed.

HOW YOU CATCH IT

BUBONIC	Usually contracted by a bite from a flea that previously fed on an infected animal. Animals that carry the bacteria, which are found in the western United States today and account for about a dozen human cases per year, are wild mice, rabbits, skunks, moles, gerbils, prairie dogs, rats, and, rarely, cats. It could also be transmitted by exposure to infected material through a break in the skin.
PNEUMONIC	Usually contracted person-to-person from breathing in tiny bacteria-carrying droplets in the air. An infected person will spray these droplets by coughing. The bacteria could be made into a weapon in a similar way: a terrorist could spray it into the air for people to breathe in. Persons can contract PNEUMONIC PLAGUE if they have BUBONIC or SEPTICEMIC PLAGUE and the bacteria spread to the lungs.
SEPTICEMIC	This rare form is usually contracted by a bite from an infected flea (see under BUBONIC for animal carriers). BUBONIC PLAGUE may also develop into SEPTICEMIC PLAGUE if the bacteria get into the bloodstream.

ASSESSMENT OF RISK

Centers for Disease Control Rating = High Priority (Category A)

Risk of Use in an Attack

PNEUMONIC PLAGUE is the form most experts believe would be used in an attack since it is the most contagious and one of the most deadly.

The deadliest strains of the plague bacteria are located in protected laboratories, so they would be difficult to obtain. The degree of technical sophistication needed to turn the bacteria into a deliverable weapon of mass infection is very high, though governmental bioweapons programs (such as Russia's) have been able to do it.

How Dangerous Is It?

Death rate if untreated,

BUBONIC: 50–60%

PNEUMONIC: Up to 100% (even if treated, could be up to 50%)

SEPTICEMIC: Up to 100%

BUBONIC PLAGUE would be less likely to spread as it did centuries ago in the times of the great plagues since we have more sanitary urban conditions.

Since the bacteria are sensitive to sunlight, heat, and disinfectants, it is estimated that they could survive and remain infectious for only up to about an hour after delivery.

TIMELINE OF ILLNESS

BUBONIC	Symptoms usually begin 2–8 days after exposure to the bacteria. If left untreated after lymph nodes begin swelling, death could follow in 2–4 days.
PNEUMONIC	Symptoms usually begin 1–6 days after exposure. If left untreated after lungs are infected, death could follow in 1–2 days.
SEPTICEMIC	Symptoms usually begin 2–4 days after exposure. Rapid progression to multiple organ failure and death could occur within a few days.

SYMPTOMS

Early-stage illness can bring on flulike symptoms such as fever, chills, weakness, and headache. Late-stage symptoms can include a purple discoloration of the skin due to systemic disease and vasculitis (inflammation of blood vessels); blackening and death of tissue (gangrene) in the extremeties, including fingers, toes, nose, and ears; seizures; and coma.

BUBONIC	High fever; painful, enlarged, warm lymph nodes (called buboes, most often in the groin and armpits, sometimes in the neck area). Pus-filled bumps or scabs could form at the site of the flea bites.
PNEUMONIC	Fever after 2–4 days; then severe pneumonia-like symptoms with cough, chest pain, coughing up blood and phlegm, and difficulty breathing. No swollen lymph nodes if infection begins in the lungs.
SEPTICEMIC	Characterized by severe fever, petechiae (patches of red dots on the skin resulting from broken blood vessels beneath the skin), and gangrene in the extremeties may also occur. No swollen lymph nodes. Rapid progression to complete, multiple organ failure.

EMERGENCY RESPONSE

- **By all means, avoid any area where an outbreak is thought to have occurred.**
- **If you must come into contact with an infected person,** stay 3–5 feet away and wear an N95 respiratory mask. Follow these precautions until the person has completed at least 3 days of antibiotic treatment.
- **Cover your mouth and nose with cloth** (wet if possible) if an N95 mask is not available in the event of an aerosol release.
- **If you have come into contact with an infected person or other airborne release:**
  - Mucous membranes (e.g., inside your mouth and nose) should be rinsed with plenty of water.
  - Eyes should be rinsed with copious amounts of a 0.9% saline solution or water (remove contact lenses first) for at least 15 minutes.
  - Skin without cuts or abrasions should be washed with soap and water.
  - Skin with cuts should be encouraged to bleed, then placed under running water and washed thoroughly with soap and water.
- **Antibiotic treatment.** In a community experiencing a pneumonic plague epidemic, persons developing a temperature of 101°F or higher or a new cough should begin antibiotic treatment immediately. Infants developing rapid breathing should be started on antibiotics as well.

  Unprotected people who have come into contact (within 6 feet) with potential patients but are not showing symptoms should take a 7-day course of antibiotics within 7 days of exposure and be monitored for fever and cough.

  If treatment is delayed for more than 1 day after onset of the symptoms, PNEUMONIC and SEPTICEMIC PLAGUES could be fatal.
- **Spray insect repellent on exposed clothes and skin** to protect from flea bites in the event of a fleaborne outbreak in your area.

TESTING AND DIAGNOSIS

An epidemic may first appear to be an influenza outbreak. However, a large number of previously healthy people rapidly progressing from fever, cough, shortness of breath, and chest pain to severe pneumonia and death would indicate the possibility of plague (inhalation anthrax is another possibility, see Chapter 1, *Anthrax*).

There is no effective environmental warning system to detect plague bacteria sprayed into the air.

Tests needed to confirm a plague diagnosis rapidly are only available at some state health departments, the Centers for Disease Control, and military laboratories.

Cultures of blood, phlegm, or lymph node fluid would show bacterial growth after 24–48 hours in labs with automated systems, 6 days for manual systems.

If there is a strong suspicion that you are infected with plague, antibiotic therapy should not be delayed before a definitive diagnosis is made.

TREATMENT

Antibiotics are the mainstay of treatment for plague. Antibiotics of choice are: streptomycin, gentamicin,* doxycycline, tetracycline, and ciprofloxacin.

Doxycycline is the first-choice recommendation for healthy adults for **mass-population protective treatment** in the event of an outbreak (if you have not been knowingly exposed but are in the area). An alternative choice is ciprofloxacin.

A **ventilator** (breathing machine) may be necessary for patients with respiratory insufficiency.

VACCINE

A vaccine that was effective only for BUBONIC PLAGUE was discontinued in 1999. A new one is in development.

CHILDREN

- For infants, rapid breathing is an early sign of infection.
- Streptomycin or gentamicin* is recommended as the antibiotic treatment for children potentially exposed. For mass-population protective antibiotic dosages, doxycycline is recommended.
- In children under 8 years old, tetracycline or doxycycline treatment may cause discoloration of teeth. In rare cases it has caused shortened skeletal growth when given to infants. The risks of tetracycline, doxycycline, and streptomycin in very young children should be discussed with your doctor.

PREGNANCY

- Streptomycin should be avoided if possible. If no other alternative is available, use as little as possible. Can be discontinued 3 days after fever has disappeared.
- Tetracycline, doxycycline, or ciprofloxacin are generally not recommended for pregnant women. Their risks should be discussed with your doctor.
- For plague, gentamicin* is the recommended treatment for exposed pregnant women and doxycycline if gentamicin is not available. If neither is available, ciprofloxacin, then tetracycline are next best.

- In the event of mass-population exposure or as preventive medications, doxycycline or ciprofloxacin are recommended. If not available, then chloramphenicol can be used.
- Breastfeeding: Gentamicin is recommended for potential exposure and doxycycline for mass-population protective antibiotic dosages. Fluoroquinolones are the recommended alternative.

SPECIAL PRECAUTIONS

Plague is somewhat difficult to diagnose because it resembles many other diseases.

If an outbreak of pneumonic plague did occur, a quarantine of patients would be necessary to prevent further spread.

* The antibiotic gentamicin is not FDA-approved for the treatment of plague but has been used successfully and is recommended as an acceptable alternative by experts.

ENVIRONMENTAL DECONTAMINATION AND CLEANUP

- Surfaces can be decontaminated with a simple germicide, such as 1 part household bleach to 9 parts water.
- Although transmission via clothing is unlikely, contaminated clothes should be washed with a germicide solution in hot water (155°F) and dried at a high temperature.
- Populations of fleas, rats, and other animal carriers, such as stray cats and dogs, must be controlled.
- There is no need for environmental cleanup in the event of aerosolized plague since the bacteria only survive for about 1 hour.

HOW YOU CAN PREPARE

Keep on hand:
    Surgical masks
    Germicide soap and disinfectant
    Insect repellent

Keep health-facility and emergency phone numbers readily available (see *ADDITIONAL RESOURCES* below and the *Public Resources and Contact Information* section of the book).

On self-prescribing antibiotics: Unnecessary and frequent use of antibiotics could kill the weakest bacteria and leave the strongest to keep reproducing and infecting others. In this way, we could build antibiotic-resistant bacteria, or bacteria that cannot be killed by common (or possibly any) antibiotics.

Furthermore, allergic reactions to antibiotics are not uncommon and can even be life-threatening, and they may also cross-react with other medications you are taking.

ADDITIONAL RESOURCES

American College of Physicians-American Society of Internal Medicine
www.acponline.org/bioterro/plague.htm

Centers for Disease Control (CDC)
www.bt.cdc.gov/agent/plague/index.asp

Centers for Disease Control: Chemical/Biological/Radiological Hotline for obtaining information
Hotline: 888-246-2675

Centers for Disease Control: National Immunization Hotline
Hotline: 800-232-2522

National Institutes of Health
www.nlm.nih.gov/medlineplus/plague.html

National Response Center: Chemical/Biological/Radiological Hotline for reporting incidents
Hotline: 800-424-8802

State public-health locator for officials, agencies, and public hotlines
www.statepublichealth.org

The Survival Guide: What to Do in a Biological, Chemical, or Nuclear Emergency website: For updates, supplementary information, and helpful links
www.911guide.com

PLANT AND ANIMAL DISEASES

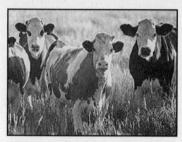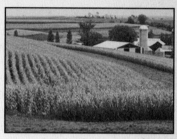

Terrorists might choose to target America's crops or livestock for many reasons, such as to make an economic impact or invoke fear in food safety.

OVERVIEW

The term "agroterrorism" refers to the use of biological weapons against animals or crops. Many experts say an agroterrorist attack would be relatively easy to perpetrate, hard to detect, and potentially disastrous economically. Though historically terrorists have used more dramatic means to get attention—usually with the spectacle of a large loss of life—agricultural terrorism has also been used. In a developing nation with limited food resources, undermining a key agricultural industry could result in widespread starvation, unemployment, civil unrest, and destabilization of government. In an industrialized nation, a response to agricultural disease would be very expensive, requiring funding to contain and decontaminate, in addition to losing profits and exports.

Reasons an Attacker Might Choose Agroterrorism
- It is relatively **"low-tech"**—for many scenarios, the level of scientific sophistication necessary to use a bacterial, viral, or chemical agent against large numbers of humans would not be required.
- There is a **lower chance of detection** by regulatory agencies due to the less regulated nature and higher accessibility of the agents that would be used.
- There is **greater personal safety to the attackers** since most agents only kill plants or animals.
- It would be **easier to deliver** since the destination would be to sparsely populated rural areas where farms are located rather than to densely populated cities.
- There is a **lower risk of large-scale, lethal retaliation** to a person, group, or rogue state.

- It **would be extremely difficult to identify the instigator,** particularly since outbreaks can occur naturally, and attackers could be far away by the time a terrorist act was detected.
- There is a **lower moral and ethical barrier to cross** (e.g., damaging the economy versus killing innocent people).

Risk of Use in an Attack

The development and weaponization of effective anti-agriculture agents would not be simple—it would require dedicated infrastructure, personnel, and resources. In order to carry out a successful agricultural attack, one would have to (1) acquire and propagate the proper biological agent, (2) process it for delivery, (3) construct an appropriate delivery device, and (4) develop a range of techniques to deal with varying weather conditions. Thus, it would require some degree of scientific sophistication.

Although the United States and other nations place export and/or trade restrictions on dangerous foreign animal and plant pathogens, it is still possible to obtain them from various international laboratories or repositories. Alternatively, pathogens can be isolated from infected animals or diseased crops. Small quantities of pathogens could easily be carried across a customs checkpoint or an unregulated border area, or sent through international mail. However, obtaining a strain of a virus or a fungus does not necessarily mean that it can be used directly as a biological weapon. For example, different strains of the rinderpest virus are similar, but they vary widely in elements such as lethality and infectability. In most cases, a terrorist would need the right strain to cause a significant disease outbreak.

In addition, if widespread destruction is the goal, moderate or high levels of scientific expertise may be needed to grow, handle, and store larger quantities of agents. Some animal pathogens are highly infectious and environmentally hardy, so processing—microencapsulation, milling, and drying—might not be necessary. But most plant pathogens and several animal pathogens are sensitive to environmental conditions; protective coatings would need to be applied to increase their chance of survival upon dissemination. Developing such coatings would involve sophisticated scientific skills that are not likely to be available to terrorists. With highly infectious pathogens, there may be no need to develop elaborate delivery devices.

Historical Incidence

The Center for Nonproliferation Studies at the Monterey Institute of International Studies maintains a database of terrorist incidents involving chemical, biological, and radiological materials perpetrated by those other than states ("substates") in the last century, and includes only 21 incidents that might be classified as examples of attacks against agriculture. Most of these 21 incidents were unsophisticated and ineffective, lacking significant impact. Only five occurred in the United States, and almost all were very small scale, involving mostly chemical rather than biological materials.

However, an effective agroterrorist attack could have an enormous economic impact, affecting revenues for years to come. Consider the apparently natural 1996 outbreak of foot-and-mouth disease among swine in Taiwan. Almost 4 million hogs were destroyed, and losses related to the swine industry were estimated to be $7 billion. Britain's battle against its mad cow disease epidemic has resulted in the destruction of about 1.5 million cattle at a cost of $4.2 billion to date and has impacted its tourism revenues as well. If this disease surfaced in the United States as it has in Britain, the economic toll could reach $15–30 billion. In fact, one-sixth of the U.S. gross domestic product and one-eighth of all jobs are either directly or indirectly connected to agriculture.

According to the Center for Nonproliferation Studies, the following states have developed or are suspected of developing biological agents against livestock and crops: Canada, Egypt, France, Germany, Iraq, Japan, North Korea, Zimbabwe, South Africa, Syria, the United Kingdom, the United States, Russia, Kazakhstan, and Uzbekistan.

NATIONAL, STATE, AND LOCAL RESPONSES TO AN ATTACK

The Animal and Plant Health Inspection Service (APHIS) and the Food Safety and Inspection Service (FSIS) are the lead agencies of the U.S. Department of Agriculture (USDA) that are charged with monitoring threats of agroterrorism. Through their field staffs, they also have developed contingency plans for dealing with emergency situations. These activities and protocols have received increased scrutiny since September 11, 2001, not unlike security procedures at airports and sporting events.

The mission of the Animal and Plant Health Inspection Service is to protect America's animal and plant resources by:
• Safeguarding resources from exotic invasive pests and diseases
• Monitoring and managing agricultural pests and diseases existing in the United States
• Resolving and managing trade issues related to animal or plant health
• Ensuring the humane care and treatment of animals

The Food and Drug Administration (FDA), which is part of the Department of Health and Human Services, is in charge of food safety as well. The FSIS handles meat, poultry, and egg inspections, and the FDA inspects everything else. The FDA and FSIS both have emergency-response units that deal with food-contamination incidents and coordinate activities with their respective field offices, the Office for Homeland Security, public-health officials, hospitals, and other federal, state, and local agencies, and sometimes foreign inspection services as well. It could take investigators time to determine whether an outbreak of foodborne illness or a crop or livestock disease was a deliberate attack, and procedures would mirror those for responding to natural outbreaks.

ZOONOTIC DISEASES

Zoonotic diseases are diseases that predominantly infect animals but can infect humans also. The following is a list of diseases covered in this book that could be used by bioterrorists against humans, animals, or both.

Disease	Animals Commonly Infected
Anthrax	Warm-blooded animals
Brucellosis	Sheep, goats, cattle, deer, elk, pigs, dogs
Glanders	Horses, donkeys, mules
Hantavirus	Rodents
Lassa Fever	Rodents
Melioidosis	Sheep, goats, horses, pigs, cattle, dogs, cats, rodents
New World Fever	Rodents
Plague	Rats, birds, pigs, wild mice, rabbits, skunks, moles, gerbils, prairie dogs, rats, cats (rarely)
Psittacosis	Birds, poultry, sheep, goats, cats
Q Fever	Livestock such as sheep, cattle, goats; household pets (rarely)
Rift Valley Fever	Sheep, cattle, buffalo, goats
Tularemia	Rabbits

LIVESTOCK DISEASES

Our Vulnerabilities

- Farm animals are vulnerable to disease since they live close together and are regularly fed antibiotics, which means they have not built up natural immunities to diseases.
- U.S. animals would be particularly susceptible to foreign diseases because they have not built up a natural resistance to them.
- Because food-processing plants are so massive, detection of the contamination of origin would be extremely difficult. For example, at a large plant that runs 20 hours per day, a single hamburger patty can contain meat from 51–1,400 cattle that originate from many different states and/or countries.
- A small outbreak could cause mass hysteria, damaging farming and food industries as well as faith in governmental safety measures.

Mad Cow Disease. Bovine spongiform encephalopathy (BSE), or mad cow disease, is a degenerative disease of the brain that affects only cattle and has infected about 1 million cows in Britain since the mid-1980s. During the final stages, infected animals become aggressive, lack coordination, and are unsteady on their hooves—hence the nickname for the condition. Since 1996, evidence has been increasing for a causal relationship between ongoing outbreaks in Europe of the disease in cattle and a disease in humans, called variant Creutzfeldt-Jakob disease (vCJD). Both disorders—caused by a transmissible agent smaller than a virus called a prion and still not entirely understood—are uniformly fatal brain diseases that can begin many years after exposure. It is believed that cattle contract the disease by ingesting feed containing contaminated meat-and-bonemeal, a protein supplement made from ground-up cattle parts. It appears that eating contaminated meat or meat products is the mode of vCJD infection in humans. Early symptoms in people are memory loss, depression, anxiety, chronic pain (especially in the feet, hands, and face), and coordination problems. Experience with this new disease is limited, but evidence to date indicates that there has never been a case transmitted person to person.

As of April 2002, a total of 125 cases of vCJD had been reported in the world: 117 from the United Kingdom, 6 from France, and 1 each from Ireland and Italy. BSE has not been detected in cattle in the United States, despite active surveillance efforts since May 1990 by the U.S. Department of Agriculture. The Centers for Disease Control monitors the incidence of vCJD in the United States, of which there has been none so far.

Note that vCJD should not be confused with the classic form of CJD that is endemic throughout the world, including the United States.

Foot-and-Mouth Disease. Foot-and-mouth disease (also called hoof-and-mouth disease) is a severe, highly communicable viral disease of cattle, swine, and other cloven-hooved animals and does not affect humans. It is characterized by fever and blisterlike lesions on and in the mouth, on the teats, and between the hooves of affected animals. Many animals recover, but the disease leaves them debilitated. It also causes severe losses in the production of meat and milk. It can be spread by animals, people, or materials that bring the virus into physical contact with susceptible animals. Due to its ability to spread rapidly, and because it has grave economic as well as clinical consequences, FMD is one of the most feared animal diseases for livestock owners.

There has not been an FMD outbreak in the United States since 1929. However, the disease is known to be widespread in parts of Africa, Asia, Europe, and South America.

Other livestock diseases (all viruses) that pose an agroterror threat are: avian influenza, bluetongue, contagious bovine pleuropneumonia, lumpy skin disease, Newcastle disease, rinderpest, African swine fever, classical swine fever, swine vesicular disease, and vesicular stomatitis.

PLANT AND CROP DISEASES

Our Vulnerabilities

- Farms are not small and widely scattered across the country anymore but are consolidated and enormous. This makes us more vulnerable, as it is the equivalent of having to attack ten mom-and-pop shops in a former time versus now having to hit just one, colossal Wal-Mart.
- Because food-processing plants are so massive, detection of the contamination of origin would be extremely difficult.
- U.S. crops would be particularly susceptible to foreign diseases because they have no natural resistance to them.

Reasons Attacks Against Crops Are Harder to Carry Out Than Livestock Attacks

- Farmers are used to combating pests and diseases affecting their crops.
- Plant and crop attacks require greater technical expertise.
- The effects would be highly dependent upon weather and environmental conditions.

An attack against crops would probably be instigated by an airborne spray. Primary targets might include cereal crops (such as wheat, barley, and rye), as the Soviet Union and Iraq aimed for in the past when they developed biological agents against crops. Other likely crop targets are corn, rice, and potatoes.

ADDITIONAL RESOURCES

Animal and Plant Health Inspection Service (APHIS)
   www.aphis.usda.gov Phone: 800-601-9327
Center for Nonproliferation Studies: Agroterrorism incidents
   cns.miis.edu/research/cbw/agchron.htm
Food and Drug Administration (FDA)
   www.fda.gov
   Consumer hotline for suspected meat and poultry contamination:
   800-535-4555
   Consumer hotline for other foods: 301-443-1240
Food Safety and Inspection Service (FSIS)
   www.fsis.usda.gov
National Response Center—Chemical/Biological/Radiological Hotline
   for reporting incidents: 800-424-8802
United States Department of Agriculture (USDA)
   www.usda.gov

PSITTACOSIS

DISEASE
Psittacosis

ORGANISM RESPONSIBLE	TYPE
Chlamydia psittaci	Bacteria

HOW YOU CATCH IT

Inhalation; contact with infected bird or animal or its environment; person-to-person transmission rare, if at all

TIME FROM EXPOSURE TO ILLNESS

5–15 days

MAJOR SYMPTOMS

Fever, chills, sore throat, hacking cough, headache, muscle aches, pneumonia

EMERGENCY RESPONSE

- Leave the area immediately in the event of a known aerosol release
- Cover your mouth and nose with a cloth (wet if possible) or wear an N95 respiratory mask to protect against inhalation
- Shower thoroughly with soap and water
- Wash clothes in hot water
- Call your doctor if you think you might have been exposed
- Begin antibiotic treatment within 24 hours of exposure

TREATMENT

Antibiotics tetracycline or doxycycline

POSSIBILITY OF DEATH

Rarely fatal with appropriate treatment

VACCINE

None for people

WHAT IT IS

Psittacosis is a systemic disease that causes flulike symptoms and may lead to pneumonia. It is caused by the bacteria *Chlamydia psittaci*, one of four species of *Chlamydia* (a better-known species is the bacteria *Chlamydia trachomata*, which causes a common sexually transmitted infection). In nature psittacosis is commonly found in birds and poultry and occasionally in sheep, goats, and cats, though it may be asymptomatic. It can be passed from birds and animals to humans.

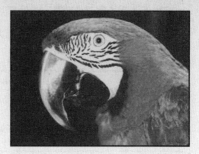

Psittacosis is also referred to as "parrot fever" because, in addition to humans and other animals and birds, it commonly infects them.

Since 1950 fewer than 50 confirmed human cases have been reported in the United States on average yearly. Although many more cases may appear that are not reported or correctly diagnosed, this low incidence suggests that if there was a widespread outbreak, it may be due to a deliberate attack.

WHAT IT DOES

Psittacosis bacteria gain entry into the body via the respiratory tract (by inhalation) and eventually harbor in the lungs and cells of the spleen, liver, kidney, heart, and occasionally the brain. An inflammatory response then takes place in the airways of the lungs, which leads to fluid-filled lung spaces where oxygen exchange normally takes place, causing obstruction of airflow. Lymph nodes in the chest become enlarged as well, and every organ where there is bacteria becomes inflamed, especially the liver and spleen.

HOW YOU CATCH IT

If psittacosis was made into an airborne spray, you would catch it by inhalation. In nature, people in contact with an infected animal would be at risk for contracting the disease. Infection is usually acquired by inhaling dried secretions from animals or birds. Occasionally the infection has resulted from contact with an environment previously inhabited by an infected bird. Person-to-person transmission occurs rarely, if at all.

ASSESSMENT OF RISK

Centers for Disease Control Rating = Second-Highest Priority (Category B)

Risk of Use in an Attack

The primary attributes of *Chlamydia psittaci* for use in a bioterror attack are that it is readily available in nature from infected birds and poultry, and it can be made into an aerosol. While the bacteria could be obtained from a place like an infected turkey farm, the search might be a long one. Additionally, quantity production of the bacteria would be difficult.

Nations, including the United States and Russia in the days of their offensive bioweapons programs (1943–1969 and 1935–1992, respectively), have investigated psittacosis for use in warfare.

Though it would be difficult to affect great numbers of people this way, it is conceivable that terrorists could infect birds or poultry as an indirect attack on humans. (To identify the infection in birds, see *SYMPTOMS* section below.)

How Dangerous Is It?

Concentrated preparations of psittacosis bacteria would easily infect humans and could be dangerous, and no effective vaccine is available. The severity of disease can range from inapparent illness to mild to severe systemic illness with pneumonia. Without proper antimicrobial treatment, theoretically 15–20% could die from psittacosis, but with treatment the number should be less than 1%. Though the disease is likely rarely spread person to person, it is difficult to predict whether widespread primary exposure would oversaturate available medical resources and result in a large number of fatalities.

TIMELINE OF ILLNESS

The time from exposure to illness would be 5–15 days. When illness begins, severe headache and fever often increase over a 3–4 day period. A dry, hacking cough may begin as late as 5 days after fever begins.

SYMPTOMS

The onset of symptoms may be subtle or abrupt and nonspecific. The most common symptoms are fever, sore throat, enlarged liver, enlarged lymph nodes, malaise, and muscle aches. Others include flulike symptoms, chills, dry, hacking cough, and headache. An enlarged spleen (splenomegaly) may be seen. Other organs that may be involved are the heart (chest pain, shortness of breath), brain (headache, seizures), skin (rash with pink spots), kidneys, and others. Abnormal clotting can occur. Gastrointestinal symptoms such as abdominal pain, vomiting, and diarrhea can also be seen. Neurologic symptoms can include lethargy, agitation, and depression, which can progress to stupor or coma in severe cases.

Symptoms in Birds

Infection among birds is called avian chlamydiosis. Whether the bird exhibits acute or chronic signs of illness or dies depends on many factors, including the species and age of the bird and the infectious dose. Signs of infection are sluggishness, ruffled feathers, nasal discharge, diarrhea, and green to yellow-green urination and droppings, and loss of appetite that could lead to emaciation, dehydration, and death.

EMERGENCY RESPONSE

- **Leave the area immediately** in the event of a known aerosol release.

- **Wearing an N95 respiratory mask** would protect against the inhalation of psittacosis organisms. If not available, cover your mouth and nose with cloth (wet if possible).

- **Shower thoroughly with soap and water.**

- **Wash clothes in hot water.** Place clothes and exposed items in sealed, double plastic bags.

- **Call your doctor** if you think you might have been exposed.

- **Begin antibiotic treatment** within 24 hours of exposure.

TESTING AND DIAGNOSIS

Diagnosis of psittacosis can be difficult. Antibiotic treatment may prevent an antibody response, thus limiting diagnosis by standard tests, and the test would not confirm infection for 4 weeks. Culture of the blood for *Chlamydia psittaci* is possible in the first 4 days of illness and from sputum in the first 2 weeks.

Psittacosis should be considered in cases of pneumonitis with splenomegaly (enlarged spleen).

Pneumonia is often evident on a chest x-ray. The x-ray, which is abnormal in 75% of patients, may not clear up for 20 weeks or more.

TREATMENT

Antibiotics of choice are tetracycline or doxycycline for 10–21 days.

In cases of severe pneumonia, a **ventilator** (breathing machine) may be required for breathing support.

VACCINE

There is a vaccine available for some farm animals.

CHILDREN

- In children under 8 years old, tetracycline or doxycycline treatment may cause discoloration of the teeth. In rare cases they have caused shortened skeletal growth when given to infants.

PREGNANCY

- In rare cases, pregnant women exposed to *Chlamydia psittaci* can contract gestational psittacosis: pneumonia, sepsis, and placental insufficiency can result in premature birth or miscarriage.
- Though tetracycline and doxycycline are recommended treatments for adults, they are not recommended for pregnant women. Consult your doctor for alternative treatments.

SPECIAL PRECAUTIONS

Use respiratory precautions (e.g., an N95 respiratory mask) if around infected birds or animals or spaces they have inhabited.

ENVIRONMENTAL DECONTAMINATION AND CLEANUP

- Since person-to-person transmission is likely rare, no isolation of patients is necessary.
- If cleaning cages of infected birds or a contaminated area, wear an N95 respiratory mask (standard surgical masks might not be protective against *Chlamydia psittaci*), protective clothing, a surgical cap, and gloves.
- Standard disinfectants should decontaminate surfaces.

HOW YOU CAN PREPARE

Keep health-facility and emergency phone numbers readily available (see *ADDITIONAL RESOURCES* below and the *Public Resources and Contact Information* section of the book).

On self-prescribing antibiotics: Unnecessary and frequent use of antibiotics could kill the weakest bacteria and leave the strongest to keep reproducing and infecting others. In this way, we could build antibiotic-resistant bacteria, or bacteria that cannot be killed by common (or possibly any) antibiotics. Furthermore, allergic reactions to antibiotics are not uncommon and can even be life-threatening, and they may also cross-react with other medications you are taking.

ADDITIONAL RESOURCES

Centers for Disease Control (CDC)
www.cdc.gov/ncidod/dbmd/diseaseinfo/psittacosis_t.htm

Centers for Disease Control: Chemical/Biological/Radiological Hotline for obtaining information
Hotline: 888-246-2675

National Institutes of Health, medical encyclopedia
www.nlm.nih.gov/medlineplus/ency/article/000088.htm

National Response Center: Chemical/Biological/Radiological Hotline for reporting incidents
Hotline: 800-424-8802

State public-health locator for officials, agencies, and public hotlines
www.statepublichealth.org

The Survival Guide: What to Do in a Biological, Chemical, or Nuclear Emergency website: For updates, supplementary information, and helpful links
www.911guide.com

U.S. Army Medical Research Institute of Infectious Diseases (USAMRIID)
www.usamriid.army.mil
Response Line: 888-USA-RIID (888-872-7443)
Questions or Comments: USAMRIIDweb@amedd.army.mil

Q FEVER

DISEASE
Q Fever

ORGANISM RESPONSIBLE	TYPE
Coxiella burnetii	Bacteria

HOW YOU CATCH IT

- By breathing in bacterial spores
- Being bitten by a tick that bit an infected animal
- By ingesting contaminated food or liquids (rare)
- Person-to-person (rare)

TIME FROM EXPOSURE TO ILLNESS

14–40 days

MAJOR SYMPTOMS

Flulike symptoms, including high fever, severe headache, fatigue, weight loss, chills, muscle pain, dry cough, sharp chest pain during inhalation, upset stomach, vomiting, and diarrhea

EMERGENCY RESPONSE

SKIN: Remove contaminated clothing and wash exposed area thoroughly with soap and water
INHALED (most likely form in bioterror attack): Cover mouth and nose with fabric (wet if possible) or wear protective N95 respiratory mask and leave vicinity, begin antibiotic treatment within 24 hours of exposure, listen for instructions from emergency management personnel regarding environmental decontamination procedures

TREATMENT

Antibiotics: tetracycline, ciprofloxacin, rifampin, doxycycline

POSSIBILITY OF DEATH

If untreated, only about 2–4%

VACCINE

Under development

WHAT IT IS

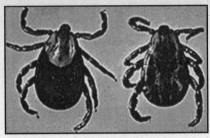

Q fever is caused by the bacteria *Coxiella burnetii* and occurs throughout the United States and world, though due to under-reporting, the incidence is unknown. It is usually found in livestock, such as sheep, cattle, goats, and (infrequently) is also found in household pets such as cats as well. It does not

Though this would be an unlikely mode of transmission in a deliberate attack, Q fever can be caught by being bitten by a tick that bit an infected animal.

usually make the animals sick; however, it will make humans sick if it is passed on to them.

When deprived of nutrients the bacteria go into a resting phase and form a hardy, protective shell around themselves called a spore. Spores allow the bacteria to resist environmental destruction and to survive for many weeks or even years. In a natural setting, infection occurs most often by people breathing in dust that has been contaminated by infected animals.

WHAT IT DOES

After being inhaled, *Coxiella burnetii* organisms multiply in lung tissue and other body organs. The bacteria enter certain immune system cells once inside the body, living in cells that usually defend us from foreign substances.

The bacteria will cause either an ACUTE form of the illness that resembles a severe case of the flu and clears up within 2 weeks (unless pneumonia develops, in which case the course could be more severe and prolonged), or a CHRONIC form that lasts for 6 months or longer, in which inflammation of the heart is the primary symptom. Rarely, Q fever may also cause liver (hepatitis), bone (osteomyelitis), or brain infection.

HOW YOU CATCH IT

- By breathing in the bacteria (or bacterial spores).
- Humans can catch Q fever from animals by breathing in dust that infected animals have contaminated or from being bitten by a tick that bit an infected animal.
- Infected tissues are highly contagious.
- Person-to-person transmission is possible but rare.

ASSESSMENT OF RISK

Centers for Disease Control Rating = Second-Highest Priority (Category B)

Risk of Use in an Attack

There are several reasons Q fever might be used in a bioterror attack:

1) The Q fever bacteria have a spore form that makes them resistant to the environment.
2) The bacteria are so infectious that even 1 bacterium inside the body can cause an infection.
3) The bacteria can be made into an airborne spray.

However, Q fever is not very lethal, which would make it undesirable for someone wishing to cause mass fatalities.

How Dangerous Is It?

Q fever is usually not a deadly disease: only about one-half of persons infected with the bacteria will show signs of illness, and most patients will return to good health within several months even without treatment. In a study of 207 untreated patients, the death rate was 2–4%.

Patients who have had heart trouble are more susceptible to the more serious, CHRONIC FORM of Q fever. As many as 65% of persons with chronic Q fever may die of the disease.

TIMELINE OF ILLNESS

The usual time from exposure to illness is about 20 days; normal range is around 14–40 days. The more bacteria taken inside the body, the shorter the time to illness will be.

Without treatment, the infection may clear up within 2 weeks. With proper antibiotics, the infection is easily treated (except for the CHRONIC FORM). If pneumonia develops, the course may be more severe and prolonged.

SYMPTOMS

The initial symptoms of Q fever are flulike, including malaise, high fever, severe headache, fatigue, weight loss, dry cough, sharp chest pain upon inhalation, upset stomach, vomiting, diarrhea, chills, sweats, confusion, body aches, and a slowed heartbeat. Pneumonia (30–50% of patients) and a certain kind of liver infection called granulomatous hepatitis (62% of patients) could develop 4–7 days after the onset of symptoms.

Q fever could also occur in a more serious, CHRONIC FORM in about 5% of patients. There may be no initial symptoms as listed above, however, a patient could experience ongoing symptoms of heart infection for 6 months to 20 years or longer. Most patients who develop this form have had a pre-existing heart condition. As many as 65% of persons with chronic Q fever may die of the disease.

EMERGENCY RESPONSE

- **Cover your mouth and nose with fabric** (wet if possible) if in the vicinity of an airborne release of the Q fever bacteria, and leave the area immediately.
- **A standard N95 respiratory protective mask** is recommended for those in the vicinity of an airborne release.
- **Antibiotic treatment.** You may be instructed to begin antibiotic treatment if there is an outbreak or attack. Antibiotic preventive treatment is most effective if started 8–12 days *after* exposure and continued for 5 days. Starting antibiotics immediately after exposure would delay symptoms but may not prevent illness.
- **Germicides.** Q fever bacteria are easily killed by disinfectants such as bleach solutions. The bacterial spores, however, are much harder to destroy. Listen for instructions from emergency management personnel regarding environmental decontamination procedures.

TESTING AND DIAGNOSIS

The symptoms of tularemia, plague, and anthrax, among other bacterial and viral illnesses, resemble those of Q fever. Laboratory testing is required to rule these out, though most laboratories do not have the facilities required for rapid, definitive testing. Confirmation can be made by determining the presence of *Coxiella burnetii* antibodies, but they are not present until 2–3 weeks after the onset of symptoms. Polymerase chain reaction (PCR) diagnostic testing is under development.

Samples for laboratory testing can be taken from the inside of the nose (with nasal swabs), or from blood, phlegm, or lung secretions.

A chest x-ray should be taken for all patients.

TREATMENT

Antibiotics of choice if infected: Tetracycline, quinolones (such as ciprofloxacin), doxycycline, or chloramphenicol. Antibiotic treatment is most effective if begun within the first 3 days of illness and should last for 2–3 weeks or until fever has subsided for 1 week. The treatment should be started again if the illness comes back. Taking the antibiotic rifampin in addition to the first-choice antibiotic has increased the effectiveness of treatment for patients who develop endocarditis (infection of the heart) or who have severe disease.

Antibiotics to protect yourself in the event of a known, widespread attack: Rifampin, tetracycline, or doxycycline. An alternative choice is ciprofloxacin. Antibiotic preventive treatment is most effective if started 8–12 days *after* exposure and continued for 5–7 days. Starting antibiotics immediately after exposure would delay symptoms but would not necessarily prevent illness.

CHRONIC Q FEVER: Doxycycline in combination with ciprofloxacin or rifampin is recommended for up 2 years.

VACCINE

A vaccine for Q fever is currently under investigation in the United States. It is licensed and available in Australia.

Persons who were previously exposed to the Q fever bacteria should not receive the vaccine due to severe reactions that could occur in the vicinity of the injection. A blood test can be done to test for the presence of antibodies against Q fever, indicating prior exposure. Those who recover fully from infection may possess lifelong immunity against re-infection.

CHILDREN

- For children over 8 years old, tetracycline for 2–3 weeks is the recommended antibiotic treatment; doxycycline is an alternative treatment (for more severe illnesses, the benefits outweigh the risks). For children under 8, trimethoprim-sulfamethoxazole (TMP/SMX, also known as Bactrim), or chloramphenicol may be recommended; for newborns up to 2 months, ciprofloxacin is prescribed. The risks of all of these drugs in infants and children should be discussed with your doctor.
- The medication recommendations above are true both for treatment of illness and for preventive treatment for a child who has been exposed and is not yet sick.

PREGNANCY

- Because the bacteria causing Q fever gravitate toward the placenta (the womb lining), pregnant women are at particular risk. Exposure of pregnant women could lead to high rates of infection of the fetus and to miscarriage.
- Treatment consists of the antibiotic combination trimethoprim-sulfamethoxazole (Bactrim), but do not take if close to the delivery date. An alternative antibiotic treatment is ciprofloxacin. The risks of these drugs should be discussed with your doctor.

SPECIAL PRECAUTIONS

See section on *PREGNANCY* above.

ENVIRONMENTAL DECONTAMINATION AND CLEANUP

- The bacterial spores are resistant to heat, drying, sunlight, and many common disinfectants.
- Decontaminate surfaces with soap and water or with a 0.5% hypochlorite solution (1 part household bleach added to 9 parts water).

HOW YOU CAN PREPARE

Wash hands regularly. As the majority of all infections are spread this way, adopting this habit will prevent everyday infections as well.

Washing clothes on a regular basis would effectively destroy the bacteria.

Keep health-facility and emergency phone numbers readily available (see *ADDITIONAL RESOURCES* below and the *Public Resources and Contact Information* section of the back). In the event of an attack, antibiotics would be most beneficial soon after exposure.

On self-prescribing antibiotics: Unnecessary and frequent use of antibiotics could kill the weakest bacteria and leave the strongest to keep reproducing and infecting others. In this way, we could build antibiotic-resistant bacteria, or bacteria that cannot be killed by common (or possibly any) antibiotics. Furthermore, allergic reactions to antibiotics are not uncommon and can even be life-threatening, and they may also cross-react with other medications you are taking.

ADDITIONAL RESOURCES

Centers for Disease Control (CDC)
    www.cdc.gov/ncidod/dvrd/qfever/index.htm
Centers for Disease Control: Chemical/Biological/Radiological Hotline
    for obtaining information
    Hotline: 888-246-2675
Centers for Disease Control: National Immunization Hotline
    Hotline: 800-232-2522
National Response Center: Chemical/Biological/Radiological Hotline
    for reporting incidents
    Hotline: 800-424-8802
National Institutes of Health, medical encyclopedia
    www.nlm.nih.gov/medlineplus/ency/article/001337.htm
State public-health locator for officials, agencies, and public hotlines
    www.statepublichealth.org

RICIN

DISEASE	
Ricin Poisoning	

ORGANISM RESPONSIBLE	TYPE
Ricinus communis	Toxin made from a plant

HOW YOU GET EXPOSED

Inhalation, ingestion, or injection

TIME FROM EXPOSURE TO ILLNESS

2–8 hours

MAJOR SYMPTOMS

INHALATION: Abrupt onset of fever, chest tightness, cough, shortness of breath, nausea, joint pain, increasingly severe breathing difficulties

INGESTION: Abdominal pain, nausea, vomiting, and profuse bloody diarrhea

EMERGENCY RESPONSE

- Cover mouth and nose with fabric (wet if possible)
- Wear tight-fitting protective N95 respiratory mask if at risk of exposure or during release if you have one
- Leave the vicinity of release immediately
- Try to hold your breath until out of the area or take shallow breaths if necessary
- Wash body, clothes, and surfaces with soap and water and/or mild bleach solution if exposed
- Listen for instructions from emergency management personnel regarding environmental decontamination procedures

TREATMENT

None, other than activated charcoal for ingested ricin

POSSIBILITY OF DEATH

If a large enough dose, most die within 28–72 hours after symptoms begin

VACCINE

Experimental only

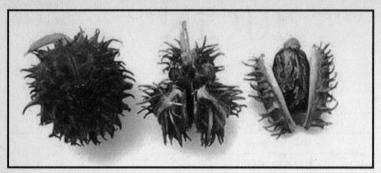

*Ricin is a toxin made from the seeds found within the beans of a castor bean plant (*Ricinus communis*), shown here.*

WHAT IT IS

Ricin is a deadly toxin derived from the castor bean plant (*Ricinus communis*). After the oil has been removed from the bean—which is used therapeutically for lubricating and laxative effects as well as in anticancer drugs—the toxin can be collected from the leftover bean mash. Ricin can be dispersed as an aerosol, liquid, or powder.

WHAT IT DOES

Ricin blocks the manufacture of vital proteins in cells, thus eventually killing the cells and causing widespread symptoms. The clinical picture depends upon the mode of toxin entry into the body.

INHALED: Affects primarily lungs, destroying lung tissue and causing the lungs to fill with fluid, leading to respiratory failure. Inhalation is the most toxic route of exposure.
INGESTED: The gastrointestinal system is affected; lesions form along the gastrointestinal tract as if by caustic burns, causing tissue death in the stomach, liver, spleen, and kidneys, then vascular collapse and death.
INJECTED: Multiple organ failure, vascular collapse, and death.

HOW YOU GET EXPOSED

Ricin is not contagious, however it would be a "convenient" terrorist agent because it could be produced as a liquid, crystal, or powder. It could be aerosolized and made into an airborne spray and INHALED, mixed into food or water and INGESTED, or as a liquid, INJECTED. Unless it is combined with an agent that would enhance absorption, absorption of ricin through the skin would be minimal.

ASSESSMENT OF RISK

Centers for Disease Control Rating = Second-Highest Priority (Category B)

Risk of Use in an Attack

Ricin may be a weapon of choice because of its high toxicity and stability, in addition to the low requirements of scientific knowledge, skill, equipment, and financial resources necessary to produce it. Further, castor beans are ubiquitous worldwide and unregulated, so the toxin is quite accessible. However, it would have to be produced in vast quantities to be used on a large scale.

Large municipal water supplies do not pose a high risk, since the toxin would not endure water-treatment processes such as chlorination, and the amount needed to produce and deliver to a reservoir would be enormous. It could be used as an airborne spray, as it would be stable as an aerosol.

Injected ricin is only a threat on very small scale; it has been used in assassinations and attempted murders.

How Dangerous Is It?

With a large enough dose, most die between 28–72 hours after symptoms begin.

TIMELINE OF ILLNESS

The timeline of both illness and lethality depend upon how much ricin a person is exposed to.

INHALED: Within an estimated 4–8 hours of inhaling aerosolized ricin particles, victims will experience severe breathing difficulties that could lead to respiratory failure in 36–72 hours.
INGESTED: Lesions, like those caused from caustic burns, emerge along the gastrointestinal tract around 2 hours after exposure. Symptoms such as vomiting and diarrhea will follow. Even if the patient is without any symptoms for 1–5 days, systemic toxicity may occur 2–5 days after exposure.
INJECTED: Symptoms could begin 36 hours after injection. Death could follow within 3 days. (Limited data.)

SYMPTOMS

INHALED: Abrupt onset of fever, chest tightness, cough, shortness of breath, nausea, joint pain, increasingly severe breathing difficulties, leading to respiratory failure. (Note that this list is based on limited data, primarily animal studies.)

INGESTED: Abdominal pain, nausea, vomiting, and profuse bloody diarrhea. In severe cases a patient may go into shock. Complications can include liver, central nervous system, kidney, and adrenal gland damage.

INJECTED: Tissue would die in the area where the needle was inserted. Symptoms would likely begin with fever, rapid heartbeat, and swollen lymph nodes; death within 3 days could occur due to systemwide collapse.

EMERGENCY RESPONSE

- **Cover your mouth and nose with fabric** (wet if possible) if in the vicinity of an airborne release of ricin, and leave the area immediately. Or, if you have one, use of a protective N95 respiratory mask is currently the best protection against inhalation. If you have to breathe before you leave the release site, take shallow breaths.

- **Unless it inhibits your escape, try to keep your eyes closed** if you are knowingly being exposed, as it is not known if the toxin can gain entry through eyes.

- **In case of aerosol attack, remove exposed clothing and seal in double plastic bags** if you believe you have been exposed. Wash clothes in bleach and hot water or have them professionally cleaned.

- **Call your doctor if you think you have been exposed.** You may be advised to go to a healthcare facility for treatment.

- **Shower as soon as possible** or wash with lots of soap and water.

- **A weak bleach solution** (0.1% sodium hypochlorite, 1 part household bleach added to 49 parts water) can be used to detoxify skin. Bleach has been shown to inactivate these compounds, but since copious amounts of water are also effective, time should not be wasted attempting to formulate bleach solutions. Never put bleach in the eyes.

- **A 10% bleach solution soak for 10–30 minutes can be used to decontaminate exposed surfaces** and articles such as jewelry, glasses, wigs, and hearing aids. Rinse with water afterward. Decontamination should be done by trained professionals; listen for instructions from emergency management personnel.

TESTING AND DIAGNOSIS

Acute lung injury affecting a large number of geographically clustered people should cause suspicion of an aerosol attack with ricin. Diagnosing ricin poisoning would mean ruling out many other biological or chemical agents that cause similar lung damage, such as anthrax, Q fever, tularemia, and phosgene. Important indicators would be that (1) ricin would likely become fatal within a few days—longer than a chemical attack such as nerve gas, yet sooner than most bacterial or viral illnesses, and (2) antibiotics would not relieve symptoms.

Once medical assistance becomes available, these laboratory tests may be helpful in the diagnosis of ricin exposure:
- Analysis of blood and respiratory secretions for the presence of ricin antigen (a very difficult test to perform)
- Elevated white blood cell count
- Chest x-ray showing injury to both lungs
- Checking antibodies for the ricin protein (a difficult test to perform and not widely available)

TREATMENT

No antitoxin treatment or other medication exists for ricin, so all treatments are supportive. These may include:

INHALED:
- **Breathing support**, such as oxygen or mechanical ventilation (breathing machine). **Raising blood pressure** with intravenous fluids and vasopressor medications. **Treatment for fluid in the lungs.**

INGESTED:
- **Vigorous pumping** and lavage (cleaning out) of the stomach.
- After lavage, **activated charcoal** may be give if the victim is conscious and alert, though it may have little value for large molecules such as ricin.
- **Fluid replacement** from fluid loss due to vomiting and diarrhea. This should be done intravenously at a hospital or clinic. Death may be avoided by early and aggressive fluid and electrolyte replacement.

VACCINE

Although there is currently no vaccine available for human use, immunization appears promising in animal models.

CHILDREN

No special precautions.

PREGNANCY

No special precautions.

SPECIAL PRECAUTIONS

When ricin is ingested, it is extremely important to keep the patient properly hydrated. Fluids should be replaced intravenously at a hospital or clinic and could mean the difference between life and death.

Although exposure to a person with ricin poisoning should generally not be a danger to others, standard respiratory and contact precautions (e.g., face mask, surgical gown, and gloves) should be taken by medical and emergency personnel coming into contact with exposed people.

ENVIRONMENTAL DECONTAMINATION AND CLEANUP

Ricin is inactivated by bleach (hypochlorite) solutions. It is also detoxified by heat (175ºF for 10 minutes). Environmental cleanup should be performed by trained professionals.

HOW YOU CAN PREPARE

Have on hand:
>   Protective N95 respiratory mask
>   Activated charcoal

Keep health-facility and emergency phone numbers readily available (see *ADDITIONAL RESOURCES* below and the *Public Resources and Contact Information* section in the book).

ADDITIONAL RESOURCES

American College of Physicians-American Society of Internal Medicine
>   *www.acponline.org/bioterro/biotoxin.htm*

Centers for Disease Control: Chemical/Biological/Radiological Hotline
>   for obtaining information
>   Hotline: 888-246-2675

Centers for Disease Control: National Immunization Hotline
>   Hotline: 800-232-2522

National Response Center: Chemical/Biological/Radiological Hotline
>   for reporting incidents
>   Hotline: 800-424-8802

State public-health locator for officials, agencies, and public hotlines
>   *www.statepublichealth.org*

U.S. Army Medical Research Institute of Infectious Diseases (USAMRIID)
>   *www.usamriid.army.mil*
>   Response Line: 888-USA-RIID (888-872-7443)
>   Questions or Comments: USAMRIIDweb@amedd.army.mil

SMALLPOX

DISEASE
Smallpox

ORGANISM RESPONSIBLE	TYPE
Variola major	Virus

HOW YOU CATCH IT

Person-to-person, usually from airborne droplets such as from an infected person coughing (or even breathing); contact with skin sores, secretions, and contaminated clothing and bedding of a patient

TIME FROM EXPOSURE TO ILLNESS

7–17 days (average is 12 days)

MAJOR SYMPTOMS

Flulike symptoms, fever, vomiting, body aches, physical exhaustion; then deep, pus-filled bumps develop on face and body (most densely on the face and limbs); unlike chickenpox, where pustules develop quickly and form and scab over at different times, smallpox bumps evolve more slowly and all form and scab over at the same time

EMERGENCY RESPONSE

– Stay away from outbreak area
– Use a respiratory mask to protect against inhaling the virus
– If there has been an aerosol release and no respiratory mask is available, cover mouth and nose with fabric (wet if possible)
– If exposed, place clothing and items touched in double plastic sealed bags; wash body thoroughly with soap and water, rinsing the inside of the mouth and nose with water; flush eyes with water or saline; and contact physician or health official immediately to obtain vaccination

TREATMENT

You can be vaccinated up to 4 days after exposure; no proven treatment later

POSSIBILITY OF DEATH

30% for untreated patients

VACCINE

Exists, but currently not available to public unless emergency situation (may be made available soon on a voluntary basis)

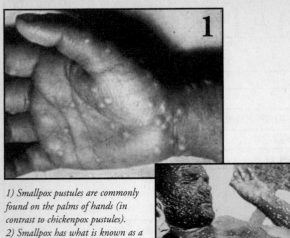

1) Smallpox pustules are commonly found on the palms of hands (in contrast to chickenpox pustules).
2) Smallpox has what is known as a centrifugal distribution—that is, the rash is denser on the face, arms, and legs than the center, or torso. In severe cases, the pustules may be extremely dense on the face and cover it entirely.

WHAT IT IS

Smallpox is a highly contagious and deadly infection caused by the virus *Variola major* (there is also a less serious form called *Variola minor*). While smallpox has killed hundreds of millions of people throughout history—as recently as the 1950s it killed 50 million a year worldwide—the virus no longer exists in nature. Hence, if even one case of smallpox was to reappear, it would most certainly be due to a bioterror attack.

WHAT IT DOES

After the virus particles are inhaled, they travel from the lungs to the lymph nodes, where they multiply. From there they travel through the bloodstream to the spleen, liver, and bone marrow, where they multiply once more. About a week later they spread to mucous membranes, such as the lining of the mouth, and then to the skin, which causes a dense rash of pus-filled, pimplelike bumps on the face and body.

HOW YOU CATCH IT

The smallpox virus is usually transmitted from person to person in airborne droplets. The reason the disease is so contagious is because an infected person develops small sores with viral particles in them in his mouth and throat, so whenever he coughs or sneezes, he is spraying virus particles into the air. Even ordinary talking and breathing can disperse particles. Persons who have come within 6 feet of an infected person are considered potentially infected. Smallpox can also be caught by coming into contact with the skin sores or secretions of a patient. **A person can pass the disease on to someone else—via air or direct contact—from the onset of the rash through its first 7–10 days.** As scabs form, infectivity decreases.

Transmission is possible via clothing and bedding as well. There are no known insect or animal carriers.

ASSESSMENT OF RISK

Centers for Disease Control Rating = High Priority (Category A)

Risk of Use in an Attack

The availability of smallpox is very low since (1) the disease has been eradicated in the world since 1977, (2) there are no natural sources, and (3) it is too large and complex a virus to be made *de novo* (from scratch), even in the most sophisticated of laboratories. However, the virus still exists in at least two authorized laboratories: one in Atlanta at the Centers for Disease Control, and one in Koltsovo, Russia (the World Health Organization inspects both frequently and has stringent safety and security precautions in place). It is not known if any other countries or groups have secret stashes; it is suspected that some nations with bioterror programs, such as Iraq and North Korea, may have gained access to the virus.

It would also be technologically difficult, although not impossible, to formulate the smallpox virus into an effective airborne spray to create a mass infection. The greatest fear is that—in our modern, mobile, unvaccinated society—a few cases could quickly spread worldwide.

How Dangerous Is It?

The death rate for *Variola major* is estimated to be 30% among the unvaccinated. For *Variola minor* it is about 1%.

While smallpox is highly contagious, one study published in December 2001 by Meltzer *et al.* in *Emerging Infectious Diseases* is somewhat optimistic in our ability to achieve containment of an outbreak if early, appropriate vaccination and quarantine procedures were implemented. In their scenario, 100 persons are assumed to be initially infected, in addition to 3 persons infected by each initial patient (this number is higher than most actual smallpox epidemic averages; however, a lot fewer people are vaccinated these days). Based on successfully contained outbreaks and mathematical models, they recommend a quarantine/vaccination-combination program, which would take a year to complete and could result in 4,200 cases. Delays in intervention would dramatically increase the number of patients for all treatment plans.

SYMPTOMS and TIMELINE OF ILLNESS

Days 0–3: After exposure, the virus migrates to the lymph nodes and multiplies. No symptoms.

Days 3–4: Symptom-free period when the virus first enters and spreads throughout the bloodstream. It multiplies in the spleen, bone marrow, and lymph nodes.

Days 8–12: Virus re-enters the bloodstream in large quantities, causing toxemia (symptoms are fever, chills, headache, body aches, and vomiting).

Days 12–14: On about the 12th day (range is day 7–17) the patient typically presents with headache, high fever (101°F or higher), malaise, physical exhaustion, and backache. Severe abdominal pain and delirium are sometimes present. A rash first emerges as red spots on the tongue and in the mouth. These spots develop into sores and break open, spreading large amounts of the virus into the mouth and upper airway. At this time, the person becomes contagious. About the same time, a rash first appears on the skin, starting on the face and spreading to the arms and legs and then to the hands and feet. Usually the rash spreads to all parts of the body within 24 hours. As the rash appears, the fever usually falls and the person starts to feel better. Within 1–2 days the rash becomes vesicular (blisterlike bumps filled with fluid) with a dip in the center, and fever may rise again.

Days 16+: A couple of days after formation of the vesicular rash, the bumps turn pustular (pus-filled bumps that are round and hard), which lasts for around 5 days. Crusts begin to form on the 8th or 9th day from the time that the rash first began, and fever will fall again. Crusts fall off after 1–2 weeks, and pitted scarring of the skin remains.

MALIGNANT FORM: A severe, highly contagious, malignant form of smallpox develops in 5–10% of patients and is often fatal within 5–7 days. The bumps are flat and not pus-filled and are so close together that the skin resembles crepe rubber. If the patient survives, the bumps will not scab over and scar; in severe cases the skin will peel away. Immune-deficient persons may be more susceptible.

HEMORRHAGIC SMALLPOX: In this very deadly form, the time to illness is shorter, and patients have severe flulike symptoms (including acute abdominal pain) before the rash sets in. The skin develops a red tint (as if flushed), and then, instead of pustules, red dots (called petechiae) the size of a pinhead are seen in patches all over the skin. These dots are tiny blood vessels that have broken and are bleeding beneath the skin, eventually leading to bruising. This form of smallpox is usually fatal within 1 week. Immune-deficient persons and pregnant women are more susceptible.

EMERGENCY RESPONSE

- **By all means, avoid any area where an outbreak is thought to have occurred.**

- **Every moment is critical in responding to a smallpox threat.** If you think you may have been exposed, contact your physician, hospital, or health department immediately and seek professional medical care.

- **If there has been an aerosol release,** put a respiratory mask on if you have one; if not, cover your mouth and nose with fabric (wet if possible).

- **If you think you have come into contact with an infected person:**
  - Mucous membranes (e.g., inside of your mouth and nose) should be rinsed with a great deal of water.
  - Rinse eyes with copious amounts of 0.9% saline solution or water (remove contact lenses first) for at least 15 minutes.
  - Skin without cuts or abrasions should be washed with soap and water.
  - Skin with cuts should be encouraged to bleed, then placed under running water and washed thoroughly with soap and water.

- **If a household member has come down with smallpox,** all clothing, bed linens, and anything else that touched the patient must be decontaminated. Heat (285ºF for 180 minutes or 340ºF for 1 hour), steam, or a germicide such as a bleach solution (1 part household bleach and 9 parts water) can be used. Refrigeration of anything contaminated will keep the virus from causing infection but will not kill it. Sealing contaminated clothing and items in double plastic bags and destroying them is recommended.

- **Wear a respiratory mask** if you must go near a person infected with smallpox. Protective gloves and clothing should be worn if you must come into direct contact with him or her.

- **Note that individuals are not known to be contagious until a rash develops,** which is typically 12–14 days after exposure.

- **The U.S. government now has a plan to vaccinate the entire population** within 10 days of a smallpox bioterror attack.

TESTING AND DIAGNOSIS

A feature of smallpox that distinguishes it from other diseases that cause similar bumps is that all of the bumps will be in the same stage at the same time (see *SYMPTOMS AND TIMELINE* section above).

The following chart illustrates the differences between smallpox and chickenpox:

Smallpox	Chickenpox
Flulike symptoms for 2–4 days prior to rash	Symptoms begin with rash
Pus-filled bumps more dense on head, arms, and legs than torso	Pus-filled bumps distributed evenly all over body, beginning on trunk
Bumps usually form on palms and soles of feet	Bumps almost never form on palms or soles of feet
Bumps slowly evolve into pustules over 7–14 days	Bumps rapidly develop into vesicles (less than 24 hours)
Bumps go through their stages at the same time	Over the course of infection, new bumps form and scab over at different times
Bumps are painful	Bumps are itchy

Fluid from skin lesions and phlegm are the secretions of choice to sample for smallpox. Nasal swabs (a Q-tip-like swab wiped inside the nose) are used to detect whether the virus is present on surfaces inside the nose and confirm exposure; nasal swabs do not confirm that the virus has caused an infection in the body.

Definitive laboratory testing requires a highly specialized laboratory with government-regulated safety equipment and procedures in place. With the use of an electron microscope, smallpox can be identified in about an hour. However, not many laboratories are equipped with these very expensive machines.

TREATMENT

There is no specific treatment for smallpox.

Immediate **vaccination** for all people who have possibly been exposed to the smallpox virus may prevent or lessen the disease if given within 4 days of exposure. It offers significant protection against a fatal outcome.

Vaccinia immune globulin (VIG), which is made from the blood products of successfully vaccinated individuals, is given along with the vaccine to people who are at risk of experiencing vaccine-related complications. It is also given to treat severe skin reactions resulting from the vaccination.

Cidofovir is an antiviral drug that has been FDA-licensed for the treatment of smallpox, although it has only been tested on animals so far. It may be used within 1–2 days after exposure. This treatment has a risk of causing serious side effects to the kidneys and must be used intravenously. There is no evidence that cidofovir is more effective than vaccination.

Patients may require **liquids** if they become dehydrated. Electrolyte drinks are recommended, such as Pedialyte (even for adults) or Gatorade.

It is not common, but if bacterial infection occurs along with the smallpox infection, antibiotics should be given. Note that this does not affect the smallpox virus itself, as viruses do not respond to antibiotics.

People who may have been exposed to the smallpox virus must be under surveillance for 17 days for fever and rash.

VACCINE

Previous vaccination. Having been vaccinated against smallpox in the past does not necessarily mean you are still immune to the disease. Though some vaccinated people may show evidence of antibodies to smallpox 30 years later, it is not known for certain whether the vaccine protects for longer than 7–10 years. The duration of immunity of those exposed to the disease previously has never been measured.

Availability. Since the last case of smallpox in the United States was in 1949, our vaccination program ceased in 1972. By the end of 2002, however, our government should have enough vaccine for every single person in the United States. The vaccine will likely be made available to emergency personnel and health care workers by early 2003, and it will probably be made available to the public on a voluntary basis sometime after that.

Side effects. A vaccination program is not undertaken lightly, as the vaccination itself can have severe and even deadly side effects for a small percentage of people (the Centers for Disease Control estimates that around 15 of every million first-time vacinees could suffer life-threatening reactions). People being vaccinated for the second time, even if it was years ago, would probably have fewer side effects. People with cancer or being treated for cancer, or with immune system deficiencies such as AIDS, or with certain skin conditions such as eczema, or who are pregnant, are most vulnerable to severe vaccine side effects. If you have any one of these conditions, you ***must*** make your doctor aware of this before receiving a vaccination for smallpox.

Protection. Vaccination for someone who has been exposed to the smallpox virus may prevent or lessen the disease if given within 4 days of exposure. Vaccination will protect a person against smallpox infection after about 7 days from the time of the injection.

CHILDREN
- Children over 1 year of age can receive a smallpox vaccination.
- Upon vaccination, up to 70% of children will get a fever of 100°F or higher for 1–2 days, and 15–20% will have a fever above 102°F.
- Children are more susceptible to contracting smallpox than adults are.

PREGNANCY
- Pregnant women are particularly susceptible to HEMORRHAGIC SMALLPOX.
- Pregnant women are considered to be at special risk for complications after the smallpox vaccine.

SPECIAL PRECAUTIONS
Persons infected with smallpox will be quarantined for at least 17 days.

See *VACCINE* section, above, for persons at risk for severe side effects from smallpox vaccination.

Aerosolized smallpox virus is most stable at low temperatures and low humidity—hence an aerosol release would be most dangerous in the winter and early spring.

ENVIRONMENTAL DECONTAMINATION AND CLEANUP
- The basic strategy of the Centers for Disease Control is to:
  1. Identify those with smallpox.
  2. Isolate those infected to keep them from infecting others.
  3. Vaccinate the people the infected person has come in contact with and other high-risk groups.
- By the time a person becomes contagious—when the rash first appears—he or she would likely be home in bed. This would probably decrease the spread of the disease.
- *Variola* virus could probably persist for as long as 24 hours if not exposed to the UV light of sunshine.
- In high temperatures (high 80s to low 90s) and humidity (80%), the *Variola* virus would be almost completely destroyed within 6 hours. In cooler temperatures (low 50s) and lower humidity (20%), about two-thirds of the virus could survive for as long as 24 hours.

- It is believed that the smallpox virus can remain viable in fabric (e.g., clothing and bedding) for extended periods if not laundered in bleach and hot water.
- Disinfectants with hypochlorite and quaternary ammonia are effective for cleaning surfaces possibly contaminated with the smallpox virus. (Note that these chemicals could damage some furniture.)
- The virus in scabs that have fallen off of smallpox lesions has been known to persist for 3–12 weeks. One group found viable virus in a 13-year-old scab discovered on a shelf. However, since the virus is bound in the matrix of the scab, it is unlikely a person could contract the disease from one, and there is no suggestion that this has occurred in the past.
- Bodies of deceased victims should be cremated whenever possible.

HOW YOU CAN PREPARE

Wash hands regularly with soap and water. As the majority of all infections are spread this way, adopting this habit will prevent everyday infections as well.

Keep a few weeks' food supply in your home as well as any other essential items you would need for such a time span. In the event of an outbreak, you may be asked to stay inside for a few days to a couple of weeks.

Keen on hand:
- Respiratory mask
- Disinfectants

Keep health-facility and emergency phone numbers readily available (see *ADDITIONAL RESOURCES* below and the *Public Resources and Contact Information* section of the book).

ADDITIONAL RESOURCES

American College of Physicians-American Society of Internal Medicine
   www.acponline.org/bioterro/index.html#smallpox
Centers for Disease Control (CDC)
   www.bt.cdc.gov/agent/smallpox/index.asp
Centers for Disease Control: Chemical/Biological/Radiological Hotline
   for obtaining information
   Hotline: 888-246-2675
Centers for Disease Control: National Immunization Hotline
   Hotline: 800-232-2522
Infectious Diseases Society of America
   www.idsociety.org/bt/toc.htm

National Institutes of Health
   www.nlm.nih.gov/medlineplus/smallpox.html
National Response Center: Chemical/Biological/Radiological Hotline
   for reporting incidents
   Hotline: 800-424-8802
State public-health locator for officials, agencies, and public hotlines
   www.statepublichealth.org
The Survival Guide: What to Do in a Biological, Chemical, or Nuclear
   Emergency website: For updates, supplementary information, and
   helpful links
   www.911guide.com
U.S. Army Medical Research Institute of Infectious Diseases (USAMRIID)
   www.usamriid.army.mil
   Response Line: 888-USA-RIID (888-872-7443)
   Questions or Comments: USAMRIIDweb@amedd.army.mil

STAPHYLOCOCCAL ENTEROTOXIN B (SEB)

DISEASE	
Staphylococcal Enterotoxin B Poisoning	

ORGANISM RESPONSIBLE	TYPE
Staphylococcus aureus	Toxin made by bacteria

HOW YOU GET EXPOSED
Ingestion or breathing it in

TIME FROM EXPOSURE TO ILLNESS
INHALED: 3–12 hours INGESTED: 4–10 hours

MAJOR SYMPTOMS
INHALED: Sudden onset of fever, headache, chills, body aches, dry cough, shortness of breath, chest pain, could lead to breathing difficulties INGESTED: Nausea, abdominal cramps, violent vomiting, diarrhea, no fever

EMERGENCY RESPONSE
INHALED (aerosol release): – Leave immediate vicinity of release site – Cover mouth and nose with cloth (wet if possible), or use a respiratory mask if available – Shower with soap and water – Wash clothes in hot water INGESTED: – Activated charcoal can be administered based on theoretical grounds, but there is no data to support its efficacy

TREATMENT
No specific treatment

POSSIBILITY OF DEATH
Probably less than 1%

VACCINE
Experimental only

WHAT IT IS

Staphylococcal enterotoxin B (SEB) is a toxin that is produced by a strain of the bacteria *Staphylococcus aureus* and is the second most common cause of food poisoning. It can live and reproduce in unrefrigerated meat, dairy, and bakery products, and it is also part of our normal body bacterial flora. If used as a biological weapon, it would most likely be aerosolized.

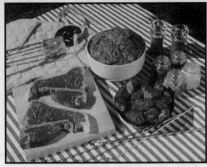

Staphylococcal enterotoxin B is a toxin that is produced by Staphylococcus aureus *bacteria and is a very common cause of food poisoning. The bacteria can live and reproduce in unrefrigerated meat, as well as in dairy and bakery products. Distributed as an aerosol, the effect of the toxin would likely be more severe than if it were ingested.*

The toxic shock syndrome toxin–1 (TSST-1), the toxin responsible for causing tampon-related toxic shock, is closely related to SEB and could cause similar symptoms if produced as an aerosol and inhaled.

WHAT IT DOES

When staphylococcal enterotoxin B enters the body, it causes an intense inflammatory response that damages tissues. The clinical syndrome depends on whether SEB is inhaled or ingested. Ingested SEB causes extreme inflammation of the gastrointestinal tract. Respiratory symptoms are due to severe inflammation of the lungs, which could cause fluid to fill the lungs and lead to respiratory failure.

HOW YOU GET EXPOSED

Staphylococcal enterotoxin B can enter the body via inhalation, eating, or drinking. Hence, it could be made into an airborne spray that would be breathed in, or it could be used to contaminate food or small-volume water supplies. It is not spread person to person.

ASSESSMENT OF RISK

Risk of Use in an Attack

Staphylococcal enterotoxin B has been investigated as a weapon of war because it could be easily aerosolized, is stable, could survive in adverse conditions, is easy to produce, and causes incapacitating illness in the majority of its victims.

How Dangerous Is It?

SEB is rarely fatal; however, it could debilitate as many as 80% of its victims for 1–2 weeks and place significant, overwhelming pressure on our healthcare system. Its effects could be much more severe if inhaled than ingested; it could lead to respiratory failure and death if inhaled at very high doses.

TIMELINE OF ILLNESS

INHALED: Symptoms begin 3–12 hours after exposure. Most patients recover in 1–2 weeks.

INGESTED: Symptoms begin 4–10 hours after ingestion, and the duration of illness is usually less than 24 hours (average is between 6–10 hours).

SYMPTOMS

INHALED: Sudden onset of flulike symptoms such as fever, headache, chills, and body aches. Respiratory symptoms include dry cough, shortness of breath, and chest pain. Nausea, vomiting, and diarrhea may also occur as a result of inadvertently swallowing the toxin. Low blood pressure may result from fluid loss. Severe inhalational exposure may cause acute lung injury (fluid filling the lungs), which may be apparent by foam coming out of the mouth or nose and could lead to respiratory failure.

INGESTED: Predominant symptoms are nausea, abdominal cramps, violent vomiting and retching, and diarrhea. Headache, weakness, and dizziness may be noted. Patients may be dehydrated, but there is generally no fever.

EMERGENCY RESPONSE

INHALED:

- **Cover your mouth and nose with a cloth** (wet if possible) and leave vicinity of aerosol release.

- **A protective respiratory mask** would be effective against toxin aerosols.

- **Shower with soap and water.**

- **Decontaminating surfaces, clothes, and objects** with a 0.5% sodium hypochlorite solution (1 part household bleach added to 9 parts water) with 10–15 minutes contact time, and/or soap and water, should inactivate the toxin.

- **Wash clothes in hot water.**

INGESTED:

- **Activated charcoal** can be administered based on theoretical grounds, but there is no data to suggest it will help.

TESTING AND DIAGNOSIS

Inhalation SEB could easily be mistaken for the flu. Suspicion of an SEB attack would arise if there were a large number of people affected in a 24–hour period, which is much less time than it would take for a naturally occurring influenza outbreak. In addition, respiratory syndromes associated with other potential bioterrorism attacks—for anthrax, tularemia, and pneumonic plague, for example—continue to progress in severity, whereas SEB would plateau rapidly. Naturally occurring ingested outbreaks can usually be tracked to a common food source.

A physical examination would probably not be helpful for the diagnosis of staphylococcal enterotoxin B.

Laboratory confirmation of SEB intoxication may involve testing blood, urine, and/or respiratory secretion samples.

Chest x-ray is usually normal, though in severe cases may show fluid in the lungs (acute lung injury).

TREATMENT

INHALED: There is no specific treatment for inhaled SEB other than **supportive**: respirator, vasopressor medication to maintain blood pressure, oxygenation, and hydration. Acetaminophen for fever and cough suppressant may also be required.

INGESTED: Staphylococcal food poisoning will usually clear up on its own within 24 hours. Vomit-inducing medication is *not* necessary. **Medication for nausea and vomiting** may relieve symptoms, such as promethazine (Phenergan), prochlorperazine (Compazine), hydroxyzine (Atarax), or trimethobenzamine (Tigan). **Antidiarrheal medications** may also be used to control diarrhea. Dehydration should be treated with **fluid replacement**.

VACCINE

There is no vaccine available at this time.

CHILDREN

Children are much more prone than adults are to suffer dangerous degrees of dehydration after bouts of vomiting and diarrhea. It might be helpful to keep oral rehydration solutions for them on hand, such as Pedialyte or sports drinks (dilute adult sports drinks with equal parts of water).

PREGNANCY

No special precautions.

ENVIRONMENTAL DECONTAMINATION AND CLEANUP

- Decontaminate surfaces with a 0.5% sodium hypochlorite solution (1 part household bleach added to 9 parts water) with 10–15 minutes contact time, and/or soap and water.
- SEB is inactivated after a few minutes at 100°F.

HOW YOU CAN PREPARE

Keep on hand:
    Respiratory masks
    Activated charcoal
    Oral rehydration solutions for children (e.g., Pedialyte)

No protective clothing is needed as SEB is not absorbed through the skin. Ordinary clothing would probably trap the toxins.

Keep health-facility and emergency phone numbers readily available (see *ADDITIONAL RESOURCES* below and the *Public Resources and Contact Information* section of the book).

ADDITIONAL RESOURCES

American College of Physicians-American Society of Internal Medicine
    www.acponline.org/bioterro/biotoxin.htm
Centers for Disease Control: Chemical/Biological/Radiological Hotline
    for obtaining information
    Hotline: 888-246-2675
National Institutes of Health
    www.nlm.nih.gov/medlineplus/staphylococcalinfections.html
National Response Center: Chemical/Biological/Radiological Hotline
    for reporting incidents
    Hotline: 800-424-8802
State public-health locator for officials, agencies, and public hotlines
    www.statepublichealth.org
The Survival Guide: What to Do in a Biological, Chemical, or Nuclear
    Emergency website: For updates, supplementary information, and
    helpful links
    www.911guide.com

T2 MYCOTOXIN ("YELLOW RAIN")

DISEASE	
T2 Mycotoxin Poisoning	

ORGANISM RESPONSIBLE	TYPE
Trichothecene mycotoxins (genus *Fusarium*)	Toxin made by fungi

HOW YOU GET EXPOSED

Absorbed through the skin, by breathing it in, or by ingestion

TIME FROM EXPOSURE TO ILLNESS

Symptoms can begin within minutes of exposure or may not start for 2–4 hours

MAJOR SYMPTOMS

SKIN CONTACT: Burning skin pain, redness, and blistering, progressing to patches of skin death and sloughing off of skin

INHALED: Nasal pain, itching, and bleeding; sneezing, runny nose, coughing, shortness of breath, wheezing, vomiting, hallucinations, mouth and throat pain with blood-tinged saliva

INGESTED: Abdominal pain, nausea, vomiting, bloody diarrhea

SYSTEMIC: Generalized weakness, dizziness, loss of coordination, low blood pressure, low body temperature

EMERGENCY RESPONSE

– Leave the area of attack immediately
– Cover your nose and mouth (with a wet cloth if possible) or wear a respiratory mask if you have one
– Do not touch people who have been in an attack
– Do not touch your eyes or other mucous membranes
– Remove outer clothing as soon as possible
– Shower with plenty of soap
– Flush eyes with copious amounts of saline or water
– Gas masks with activated charcoal filters protect against T2 inhalation; however, the use of gas masks is not recommended to the untrained due to the danger of improper use

TREATMENT

None, other than activated charcoal for ingested T2

POSSIBILITY OF DEATH

Can produce significant life-threatening disease if delivered as an aerosol

VACCINE

In development

WHAT IT IS

Trichothecene mycotoxins are a group of 40-odd different toxic compounds that are produced by fungi (molds) of the genus *Fusarium*. They are commonly found in grain and are extremely hardy in the environment. Technically known as biological agents, myco-toxins actually act more like chemical agents than bio-weapons because they are fast-acting, affect the skin and mucous membranes as well as the lungs and gastrointestinal tract, and destroy cells by

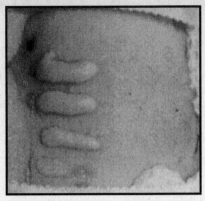

This experiment shows the blistering effects of T2 mycotoxin: Depicted here are vesicles and erosions on the back of a hairless guinea pig at 1, 2, 7, and 14 days (top to bottom) after application of a tiny amount of T2 mycotoxin mixed with methanol.

disrupting the functioning of DNA. In fact, mycotoxin is the only class of biologic toxin that can directly affect the skin.

One of the most deadly of the trichothecene mycotoxins is the T2 mycotoxin, which is about 100 times more potent than mustard gas or lewisite (see Chapters 18 and 19). T2 has reportedly been used in warfare by several countries beginning in the mid-70s. Because aircraft delivered it in the form of mostly yellow-colored smoke, dust, and sticky droplets, it came to be known as "yellow rain."

The countries that allegedly used it are Russia, Afghanistan (probably supplied by the Soviets), North Vietnam, and Laos. Iraq has admitted to testing it on animals.

WHAT IT DOES

Trichothecene toxins affect many systems of the body, the mechanisms of which are poorly understood. T2 toxin is rapidly absorbed into the lung and stomach lining and more slowly taken up through the skin. Its effect stems from its ability to quickly stop DNA function, which is vital to the functioning of cells. It mostly affects rapidly dividing cells, such as those in bone marrow, the gastrointestinal tract, skin, and reproductive cells.

T2 may also suppress the immune system, allowing for secondary, opportunistic bacterial infections to develop.

HOW YOU GET EXPOSED

T2 can be ingested, inhaled, or absorbed through the skin. Mycotoxins have been implicated in foodborne illnesses on several continents and have been hazardous to farmers and domestic animals who are exposed through contaminated dusts and hay.

ASSESSMENT OF RISK

Centers for Disease Control Rating = High Priority (Category A)

Risk of Use in an Attack

T2 mycotoxin may be selected as a bioweapon because it is extremely stable in the environment—it is exceptionally resistant to heat and sunlight (ultraviolet light) inactivation and can last for weeks. Since it is a common grain mold, it is also easily available. Moreover, production using modern fermentation methods similar to brewing or antibiotic production is fairly easy and inexpensive, and conventional bioreactors can produce tons of these agents without much difficulty. Because they are so hardy, they could be delivered by mortars, artillery, rockets, aerial bombs, and surface or aerial sprayers.

How Dangerous Is It?

T2 is about 100 times more potent than the blister agents mustard gas or lewisite, particularly in its ability to injure skin and eye tissue. T2 could produce significant life-threatening disease if delivered as an aerosol. Thousands died after the alleged yellow rain attacks of the 1970s and 1980s.

T2 could also be mixed with other agents to facilitate dispersal and handling of the toxin and to enhance its toxicity.

TIMELINE OF ILLNESS

SKIN CONTACT: Time from exposure to illness is minutes to hours.
INHALED: Time from exposure to illness is minutes.
INGESTED: Time from exposure to illness is minutes.
SYSTEMIC: After ingestion, inhalation, or skin exposure, systemic symptoms may precede eventual death by minutes, hours, or days.

SYMPTOMS

SKIN CONTACT: Symptoms begin with burning skin pain, redness, and blistering, progressing to patches of skin death and sloughing off of skin.

INHALED: Nasal pain, itching, and bleeding; sneezing, runny nose, coughing, shortness of breath, wheezing. Mouth and throat pain and blood-tinged saliva.

INGESTED: Abdominal pain, nausea, vomiting, bloody diarrhea.

SYSTEMIC: Systemic toxicity can occur via any route of exposure. Symptoms are generalized weakness, dizziness, difficulty walking, loss of strength, exhaustion, and loss of coordination, followed by low blood pressure and low body temperature. Death could occur in minutes, hours, or days once these symptoms begin.

EMERGENCY RESPONSE

- **Leave the area of attack immediately** to limit your exposure and seek fresh air.
- **Cover your nose and mouth** (with a wet cloth if possible) or wear a respiratory mask if you have one.
- **Try to keep your eyes closed** unless this inhibits your escape.
- **Do not touch people who have been in an attack. Do not touch your eyes or other mucous membranes,** as the toxin can gain entry quickly into your body this way.
- **Remove outer clothing** as soon as possible and place in double plastic sealed bags for hazardous waste disposal. Because clothing can serve as a reservoir for further toxin exposure if not decontaminated, further decontamination should be performed by professionals trained in the use of specialized solutions such as 1% hypochlorite (bleach) solution and 0.1M sodium hydroxide (NaOH).
- **Thorough washing with soap and uncontaminated water** will effectively remove this oily toxin from exposed skin and other surfaces. This can reduce toxicity to the skin even if delayed 4–6 hours after exposure.
- **Flush eyes** with copious amounts of saline or lukewarm water for 15 minutes.
- **Activated charcoal should be taken** for ingested T2.

TESTING AND DIAGNOSIS

Physical evidence such as a yellow, red, green, or other-pigmented oily liquid suggests mycotoxins. The rapidity of symptom onset would also suggest a toxin (or chemical) attack.

Differentiating T2 from other agents:
- Mustard gas and other blister agents usually have an odor and can be detected by a military field chemical test (M8 proper, M256 kit).
- Inhalation of staphylococcal enterotoxin B (SEB) or ricin aerosols can cause fever, cough, and shortness of breath but do not involve the skin.

A rapid environmental diagnostic test is not available. The presence of T2 can be confirmed in environmental or biological samples using a method called gas chromatography/mass spectrometry. Blood and urine analysis can detect antigens to T2, and T2 byproducts can be detected as late as 28 days after exposure.

TREATMENT

No antidote or specific therapeutic regimen is available for T2 poisoning, hence treatment is **supportive**, such as burn care for skin lesions. Standard therapy for poison ingestion should be administered, such as **activated charcoal** to absorb swallowed T2.

Patients should be monitored for respiratory distress. If a cough or breathing difficulty develops, patients should be evaluated for decreased oxygen levels or inflammation of the lungs or airways.

VACCINE

There is no vaccine available, but there is one under development.

CHILDREN

No special precautions.

PREGNANCY

No special precautions.

SPECIAL PRECAUTIONS

In the event of a T2 mycotoxin release, make every effort to cover your entire body in protective clothing, as T2 is absorbed through the skin, eyes, and mucous membranes.

ENVIRONMENTAL DECONTAMINATION AND CLEANUP

Trichothecene mycotoxins are very resistant to environmental degradation and can withstand heat up to 500°F. Because T2 is so hardy, it is extremely difficult to inactivate. Instead, attempts should be made to wash it away, which soap and water can do very effectively. This is effective for both skin and surfaces.

Trained professionals should perform decontamination. To inactivate the toxin, a 1% hypochlorite (bleach) solution is necessary, in addition to 0.1M sodium hydroxide (NaOH) solution, with a 1-hour contact time.

HOW YOU CAN PREPARE

Keep health-facility and emergency phone numbers readily available (see *ADDITIONAL RESOURCES* below and the *Public Resources and Contact Information* section of the book).

Note that a charcoal-activated gas mask, while protective, would likely be impractical in the event of an attack. It weighs about four pounds, and you would have to carry it everywhere to be ready for a surprise strike. If you choose to purchase one for your home, you must read the instructions carefully and practice with it, as improper use will not protect you and could actually suffocate you. WARNING: Our medical experts do not recommend the use of gas masks except by trained professionals. Data from Israel shows that the incorrect use of gas masks has caused many fatalities.

ADDITIONAL RESOURCES

American College of Physicians-American Society of Internal Medicine
www.acponline.org/bioterro/biotoxin.htm

Centers for Disease Control: Chemical/Biological/Radiological Hotline for obtaining information
Hotline: 888-246-2675

Centers for Disease Control: National Immunization Hotline
Hotline: 800-232-2522

Medical NBC Online
www.nbcmed.org/sitecontent/medref/onlineref/fieldmanuals/ medman/mycotoxins.htm

National Response Center: Chemical/Biological/Radiological Hotline for reporting incidents
Hotline: 800-424-8802

State public-health locator for officials, agencies, and public hotlines
www.statepublichealth.org

The Survival Guide: What to Do in a Biological, Chemical, or Nuclear Emergency website: For updates, supplementary information, and helpful links
www.911guide.com

U.S. Army Medical Research Institute of Infectious Diseases (USAMRIID)
www.usamriid.army.mil
Response Line: 888-USA-RIID (888-872-7443)
Questions or Comments: USAMRIIDweb@amedd.army.mil

TULAREMIA

DISEASE	
Tularemia	

ORGANISM RESPONSIBLE	TYPE
Francisella tularensis	Bacteria

HOW YOU CATCH IT

Ingesting undercooked meat or contaminated water, breathing it in, contact with infected animals or animal parts, bite from infected tick or fly

TIME FROM EXPOSURE TO ILLNESS

1–21 days (usually 3–5 days)

MAJOR SYMPTOMS

INHALATIONAL TULAREMIA (most likely form in bioterror attack): sudden onset of fever, muscle ache, malaise, sore throat, upset stomach, weakness, pneumonia with dry cough, sharp chest pain, rash, vomiting, diarrhea
SKIN (most commonly occurring in nature): open sore (ulcer) on the skin, painful swollen lymph nodes

EMERGENCY RESPONSE

INHALED:
— Leave contaminated area immediately
— Cover mouth and nose with wet cloth or wear an N95 respiratory mask if available
— Wash body and clothes thoroughly with soap and hot water
— Begin antibiotic treatment within 24 hours of potential exposure
SKIN exposed to bacteria:
— Wash immediately with soap and hot water

TREATMENT

Antibiotics such as streptomycin and gentamicin

POSSIBILITY OF DEATH

Less than 4% if treated; 33% if untreated
Mortality rate of pulmonary tularemia may be as high as 60%

VACCINE

Under review by FDA, may be available in the future

WHAT IT IS

Also known as rabbit fever and deerfly fever, tularemia is an extremely contagious disease that is usually found in animals and is caused by the bacteria *Francisella tularensis*. Only 10–50 of the microscopic organisms are necessary to cause an infection.

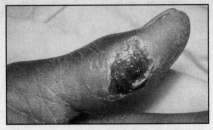

A skin ulcer shows up in the majority of tularemia patients infected naturally. Ulcers are generally single lesions with heaped up borders 1/4 – 1-1/4" in diameter. A bioterror attack would likely be aerosolized and breathed in, however, and thus not produce an ulcer.

The bacteria are found naturally in soil, water, and vegetation in rural areas. They can remain alive for weeks in water, soil, and animal hides and carcasses. In cold, moist conditions they can survive for months, and they have been known to remain infectious in frozen rabbit meat for years.

The type of tularemia that a person comes down with usually depends upon how the bacteria enter the body. The two most severe forms— PNEUMONIC TULAREMIA and TYPHOIDAL TULAREMIA—can be caused by breathing in the bacteria. There have only been about 200 cases of tularemia reported in the United States in the last decade, and of those, only about 5% were the inhaled varieties. Thus, if an outbreak of inhalational tularemia occurred, it would very likely be due to a biological attack.

WHAT IT DOES

Once inside the body, tularemia bacteria multiply inside certain specialized white blood cells of the immune system that normally act to kill our body's foreign invaders. This allows the bacteria to freely grow and spread inside the body. The major targets are the lymph nodes, lungs, spleen, liver, and kidneys.

HOW YOU CATCH IT

The *Francisella tularensis* bacteria can infect humans through the skin, mucous membranes, gastrointestinal tract, and lungs. Tularemia can thus be contracted by ingesting contaminated meat or water or from breathing in bacteria that have been sprayed into the air (aerosolized). Humans can catch it from animals (such as rabbits, squirrels, deer, voles, mice, water rats, beavers, and raccoons) by coming into contact with infected animal tissue, body fluids, and pelts (fur still attached to the skin), or from bites of infected animals. It can also be caught from tick or fly bites.

ASSESSMENT OF RISK

Centers for Disease Control Rating = High Priority (Category A)

Risk of Use in an Attack

Though found in animals in nature, the bacteria causing tularemia would be difficult to process as a weapon. They are also not very stable and are killed by mild heat and disinfectants. However, because tularemia bacteria are so infectious, if someone could engineer them to be delivered effectively, especially in an airborne fashion that would not destroy them, most of those exposed would become infected.

How Dangerous Is It?

If untreated, tularemia is fatal in 33% of cases. In cases involving the lungs and other organ systems, the death rate may rise to 60%. With adequate antibiotic treatment for 10–14 days, however, almost everyone rapidly improves.

TIMELINE OF ILLNESS

Onset of illness after exposure is usually between 3–5 days but can be anywhere from 1–21 days.

Treatment in the early stages usually results in complete recovery. Untreated tularemia could persist for several weeks or months, usually with increasing symptoms and bodily weakness.

SYMPTOMS

There are many types of tularemia. Spraying the bacteria in the air, as would likely be the case in a bioterror attack, would cause INHALATIONAL (PNEUMONIC) TULAREMIA. Major symptoms in this syndrome are:

- Sudden onset of fever, headache, chills, muscle ache (especially in the lower back), malaise, sore throat, shortness of breath, chest discomfort, potentially life-threatening pneumonia with dry cough (no production of mucus or blood), and 30% of patients will develop a rash. Upset stomach, vomiting, and diarrhea may sometimes occur. The infection could enter the bloodstream and become systemic (spreading throughout the entire body).
- As the illness continues, patients will also have sweats, weight loss, and progressive weakness.

A tularemia throat infection (OROPHARYNGEAL) could be caught from inhaling contaminated droplets in an aerosolized spray. Patients would develop a severe sore throat and sometimes tonsillitis with ulcers. Swollen lymph nodes may occur.

TYPHOIDAL TULAREMIA is a deadly form of the disease and is used to describe a systemwide illness when no clear source of organism entry is found. These patients sometimes exhibit prominent intestinal symptoms, such as diarrhea and abdominal pain, in early stages of the disease. It can result in organ and respiratory failure if not caught and treated in time.

Although these forms are unlikely to occur in an aerosol bioterror attack, tularemia can also infect the skin (ULCEROGLANDULAR, most common in nature, causing an open sore on the skin), eyes (OCULO-GLANDULAR), stomach (GASTROINTESTINAL), and brain (MENINGEAL).

EMERGENCY RESPONSE

- **Avoid any area where an outbreak is thought to have occurred.**
- **After an airborne release,** cover mouth and nose with a wet cloth or an N95 respiratory mask if available.
- **Wash thoroughly with soap and water.** This is extremely important since such a small amount of bacteria is necessary to cause infection (10–50 organisms).
- **Clothes can be decontaminated by washing with soap in hot water,** as heat kills the bacteria.
- **In the event of food or water contamination,** cook food thoroughly or boil water.
- **Keep an eye on the health of family pets such as cats and dogs.** Since tularemia can be passed to humans from animals, it is possible they could contract it and pass it on to you. Call your local veterinarian if you suspect your pet has tularemia.

TESTING AND DIAGNOSIS

Tularemia is difficult to diagnose because it is so similar to other illnesses. Further, there is no widely available, rapid test to diagnose it (rapid antibody testing is a diagnostic procedure performed only in designated reference laboratories). For this reason it is recommended that a diagnosis be made based primarily on symptoms alone, particularly in the event of a known outbreak. A large number of cases at the same time of high fever and pneumonia with dry cough would be consistent with a bioterror attack of tularemia.

The *Francisella tularensis* bacteria can be recovered from lung fluid, lymph nodes, wounds, phlegm, stomach secretions, and blood (rarely) and tested. A chest x-ray could also be taken.

TREATMENT
Antibiotics of choice if infected: Streptomycin would be the first choice, or gentamicin. Ciprofloxacin has also been found to be effective against tularemia. A combination of streptomycin and a third-generation cephalosporin should be used for TULAREMIA MENINGITIS (infection of the brain or spinal cord lining). Oral antibiotics that can be used are doxycycline, tetracycline, and ciprofloxacin.

Those who are knowingly potentially exposed and come down with fever and flulike symptoms within 14 days of exposure should begin antibiotic treatment. It is important to be evaluated by your doctor. If you think you might have been exposed and have not taken antibiotics, monitor yourself for fever several times a day; seek medical care immediately if your temperature reaches 100°F.

Antibiotics to protect yourself in the event of a known, widespread attack: Doxycycline, tetracycline, and ciprofloxacin. If you start treatment within 24 hours of exposure you may avoid symptoms of the disease. If you take antibiotics before you become ill as a preventive measure, continue taking them for 14 days.

A mechanical breathing machine (**ventilator**) could be necessary if your breathing is impaired.

VACCINE
In the past there was a vaccine available for lab workers who routinely used the tularemia bacteria, but it is currently under review by the Federal Drug Administration (FDA). The vaccine does not work if given after exposure.

CHILDREN
- Antibiotics of choice are streptomycin or gentamicin. Doxycycline and ciprofloxacin could be given orally. While there are usually precautions for these drugs for young children, the benefits outweigh the risks in this case; the risks of these drugs should be discussed with your doctor.

PREGNANCY
- Antibiotics of choice are gentamicin or streptomycin. Doxycycline and ciprofloxacin are alternative choices. While there are usually precautions for these drugs for pregnant women, the benefits outweigh the risks in this case; the risks of these drugs should be discussed with your doctor.

ENVIRONMENTAL DECONTAMINATION AND CLEANUP
- Quarantine is not necessary since tularemia is not spread from person to person.

- Tularemia bacteria are easily inactivated by mild heat (55°F for 10 minutes) and/or standard disinfectants such as a 0.5% sodium hypochlorite solution (1 part household bleach added to 9 parts water).
- Clothing or linens with body fluids of patients with tularemia should be washed with disinfectant.

HOW YOU CAN PREPARE

Purchase a protective N95 respiratory mask. Wearing this could prevent contracting the disease if the bacteria were sprayed into the air in your vicinity.

Keep health-facility and emergency phone numbers readily available (see *ADDITIONAL RESOURCES* below and the *Public Resources and Contact Information* section of the book). In the event of an attack, antibiotics would be the most effective treatment in combating tularemia if taken within 24 hours of exposure.

On self-prescribing antibiotics: Unnecessary and frequent use of antibiotics could lead to the production of antibiotic-resistant bacteria. In addition, allergic reactions to antibiotics are not uncommon, and they can cross-react with other.

ADDITIONAL RESOURCES

American College of Physicians-American Society of Internal Medicine
  www.acponline.org/bioterro/tularemia.htm
Centers for Disease Control (CDC)
  www.bt.cdc.gov/agent/tularemia/index.asp
Centers for Disease Control: Chemical/Biological/Radiological Hotline
  for obtaining information: 888-246-2675
Centers for Disease Control: National Immunization Hotline
  Hotline: 888-232-2522
Federal Drug Administration (FDA)
  www.fda.gov
National Institutes of Health, medical encyclopedia
  www.nlm.nih.gov/medlineplus/ency/article/000856.htm#prevention
National Response Center: Chemical/Biological/Radiological Hotline
  for reporting incidents: 800-424-8802
State public-health locator for officials, agencies, and public hotlines
  www.statepublichealth.org
Tularemia as a Biological Weapon
  www.jama.ama-assn.org/issues/v285n21/ffull/jst10001.html#a11

VIRAL HEMORRHAGIC FEVERS

DISEASES

Ebola Hemorrhagic Fever, Marburg Hemorrhagic Fever, Lassa Fever, New World Hemorrhagic Fever, Rift Valley Fever, Hantavirus Infection, and Yellow Fever

ORGANISMS RESPONSIBLE

There are four major families of viral hemorrhagic fevers (VHFs): filoviruses (Ebola and Marburg), arenaviruses (Lassa, New World), bunyaviruses (Rift Valley, hantavirus), and flaviviruses (yellow)

TYPE

Virus

HOW YOU CATCH THEM

These diseases are usually caught via a bug bite or from direct contact with an infected person or animal or their secretions; people would become infected after an aerosolized attack by breathing the virus into their lungs or from mucous membrane (eyes, mouth, and lining of nose) exposure

TIME FROM EXPOSURE TO ILLNESS

Approximately 2–21 days

MAJOR SYMPTOMS

Fever; headache; muscle aches; extreme weakness; eye inflammation; rash; low blood pressure; bruising; bleeding from the eyes, mouth, nose, and/or gastrointestinal tract; kidney failure; confusion

EMERGENCY RESPONSE

- For an airborne release of a VHF virus, cover your mouth and nose with fabric (wet if possible) or a respiratory mask; remove clothes and place in double plastic sealed bags; wash body thoroughly with soap and water (shower if possible); rinse out eyes, nose, and mouth
- Limit contact with infected persons
- Immediately wash with soap and water any part of your body (shower if possible) exposed to blood, body fluids, secretions, or excretions from patients with suspected VHF infection
- Protective clothing and a powered air-purifying respirator (or respiratory mask) should be worn around patients who are coughing, vomiting, bleeding, or have diarrhea
- Thoroughly decontaminate any object, clothing, or material an infected person has come in contact with

TREATMENT

No proven treatment, though the antiviral drug ribavirin may be helpful in some cases

POSSIBILITY OF DEATH

EBOLA: 50–90%	MARBURG: 25–70%	LASSA: 15–20%	NEW WORLD: 15–30%
RIFT VALLEY: Less than 1%	HANTAVIRUS: 1–15%	YELLOW FEVER: 20%	

VACCINE

Available for YELLOW FEVER only

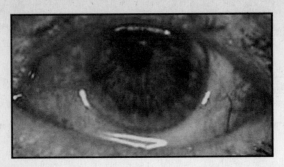

A cardinal sign of viral hemorrhagic fevers is reddened and inflamed mucous membranes of the eyes (conjunctiva).

WHAT THEY ARE

Viral hemorrhagic fevers (VHFs) are a group of diseases caused by different viruses that produce similar effects: high fever and other flulike symptoms and widespread bleeding, which can be extensive throughout the body, both internally and externally. The diseases that will be discussed in this chapter are EBOLA, MARBURG, LASSA, NEW WORLD, RIFT VALLEY, HANTA, and YELLOW VIRAL HEMORRHAGIC FEVERS, which are among the primary VHFs that the Centers for Disease Control has cited as being the most likely to be made and used as weapons.

Natural Incidence of Disease

EBOLA: There have been four known outbreaks of Ebola hemorrhagic fever since its initial recognition in 1976 (two in Sudan and two in Zaire). There have been no confirmed cases in the United States.

MARBURG: Isolated cases have occurred in Africa. Outside of Africa two small outbreaks are known (one in Germany and one in Yugoslavia, both in 1967) but were linked to sources in Africa. There have been no confirmed cases in the United States.

LASSA: Lassa fever is found mainly in West Africa, where the number of infections per year is roughly estimated to be 100,000–300,000, with approximately 5,000 deaths.

NEW WORLD: Outbreaks are rare and have primarily occurred in South American countries (Argentina, Bolivia, Venezuela, Brazil). There has never been an outbreak in the United States.

RIFT VALLEY: Occasional outbreaks have occurred affecting large numbers of people; these have usually been confined to Africa, although an outbreak in 2000 occurred in Saudi Arabia and Yemen.

HANTAVIRUS: Approximately 150,000–200,000 cases of hantavirus hemorrhagic fever involving hospitalization are reported each year throughout the world. More than half of those are reported in China, and Russia and Korea report hundreds to thousands of cases each year as well. YELLOW FEVER: There are 200,000 estimated cases of yellow fever (with 30,000 deaths) per year, with the large majority being from central Africa. In the Americas, yellow fever is endemic in nine South American countries and in several Caribbean islands. There has not been an outbreak in the United States since 1905.

WHAT THEY DO

The term "hemorrhagic" refers to the virus's ability to cause blood vessels to rupture and hemorrhage, or bleed, which in turn causes blood to leak under the skin, in internal organs, and from the mouth, nose, eyes, or other body openings. Although most patients develop significant bleeding and bruising, the bleeding itself is rarely life-threatening. More significantly, the overall vascular system is damaged, impairing the body's ability to regulate itself; thus, the most fatal aspects of these diseases are dwindling blood pressure and shock. For some of the VHFs it seems that the virus also affects blood clotting factors (which normally enable a wound to stop bleeding) and the immune system. Limited data exist since the diseases are so rare in humans.

HOW YOU CATCH THEM

The infectious stage for VHFs appears to be after the patient or animal develops symptoms.

In nature, VHFs are usually transmitted to humans from contact with infected animals—usually rodents—or from the bite of a bug carrier such as a spider, mite, or tick. In most cases the virus can get into the body through mucous membranes like the mouth, lining of the nose, and eyes. Because EBOLA, MARBURG, and LASSA viruses are present in the skin cells and sweat glands, these forms can be caught by touching an infected person or corpse.

The animal or insect hosts or reservoirs where the EBOLA and MARBURG viruses exist in nature are unknown; it appears that the viruses are passed on by direct or close contact with infected people and nonhuman primates or their bodily secretions/excretions. LASSA FEVER, NEW WORLD, and other ARENAVIRUSES can be contracted by direct contact with infected blood or secretions or by inhaling particles that become airborne from infected rodent urine or droppings. RIFT VALLEY FEVER is usually caught from a mosquito bite, from contact with infected tissue, urine, or droppings, or from inhaling the virus particles coming from dead infected animals, or possibly from ingesting uncooked milk from infected animals. Susceptible livestock are sheep, cattle, buffalo, and goats. HANTAVIRUSES are known to be carried by certain rodents; it appears that the infection may be caught by direct or close contact with the infected rodents or their bodily secretions/excretions as well as by inhaling particles that become airborne from infected rodent urine or droppings. The usual route of transmission of YELLOW FEVER is by mosquito bite.

Person-to-person transmission of the viruses from airborne droplets (carried in the air when an infected person coughs, talks, or breathes) may be possible.

ASSESSMENT OF RISK

Centers for Disease Control Rating = High Priority (Category A)

Risk of Use in an Attack

VHFs have been studied in several government-sponsored bioweapons programs as recently as 1992. All of the viruses listed in this chapter could potentially be engineered into an aerosolized weapon. In addition to developing the virus into a spray that could be delivered, for example, via a crop-duster airplane or through the ventilation system of a building, it is theoretically possible that these viruses could be made to infect an insect population that would in turn be set loose on a human population.

It would not require an enormous amount of technological skill to weaponize these viruses, though given how deadly the diseases are, it would be a very dangerous and possibly deadly endeavor to prepare them. The obtainability of the VHF viruses for bioterrorist use varies; some of the strains could be obtained from the natural environment (e.g., ARENAVIRUSES exist in rodents in certain parts of the world), but some, like EBOLA, would be very difficult to obtain.

How Dangerous Are They?
The viruses represent a range of potency, ranging from a less than 1% death rate (RIFT VALLEY FEVER) to up to 90% (EBOLA).

TIMELINE OF ILLNESS

In general, patients begin to show symptoms within 2–21 days. Initial symptoms are flulike and typically last less than a week. In severe cases, patients then progressively show more signs of hemorrhaging, with rashes and bleeding from the eyes, nose, mouth, and/or gastrointestinal tract.

Time from Exposure to Illness

EBOLA: usually about 1 week (2–21 days)
MARBURG: 2–14 days
LASSA: 5–16 days
NEW WORLD: 7–14 days
RIFT VALLEY: 2–6 days
HANTAVIRUS: 9–35 days
YELLOW FEVER: 3–6 days

SYMPTOMS

In general, patients with a viral hemorrhagic fever become ill first with flulike symptoms, which typically include high fever, headache, malaise, body aches, nausea, abdominal pain, and nonbloody diarrhea. Other early symptoms are low blood pressure, slowed heart rate, rapid breathing, eye inflammation, sore throat, and a rash or flushing of the skin. Although these symptoms are characteristically accompanied by significant bleeding and bruising, the bleeding itself is usually not life-threatening.

EBOLA, MARBURG, RIFT VALLEY FEVER, and YELLOW FEVER all begin with an abrupt onset of symptoms, while LASSA and HANTA FEVER symptoms emerge more gradually.

EBOLA and MARBURG: Initially patients experience flulike symptoms like fever, headache, muscle aches, joint pain, and sore throat, commonly followed by vomiting, diarrhea, and stomach pain. A peeling skin rash resembling measles (spread-out pink, solid bumps) often appears 5–7 days later. Hemorrhaging usually begins after the third day of illness and can include patches of tiny red dots on the skin (called "petechiae," these are tiny broken blood vessels just beneath the skin's surface), as well as internal and external bleeding from multiple sites. A person may have a high fever and be delirious throughout the illness. A short period without fever may come before multi-organ failure and death.

LASSA FEVER: Initially patients experience flulike symptoms very similar to EBOLA and MARBURG, including coughing without congestion. During the second week of illness, congested lungs may develop, as well as a rash of flat, hard bumps or petechiae, nervous-system abnormalities such as tremors and seizures, and bleeding from eyes and mucous membranes. Later symptoms may include severe swelling of the face and neck. Death usually results from respiratory failure and shock rather than life-threatening blood loss. In milder cases, the patient begins to recover in 2–8 days from the beginning of illness. The most common after-effect is deafness (25% of patients), even in mild cases.

NEW WORLD: Patients experience the gradual onset of fever, body aches, nausea, abdominal pain, inflammation of the conjunctiva (white surface of the eyes), flushing of the face and trunk, and swollen lymph nodes. They may develop petechiae, bleeding, and central nervous system dysfunction (tremors of the tongue and upper extremities, muscle twitches, disturbances in articulation due to incoordination of speaking muscles, and generalized seizures).

RIFT VALLEY FEVER: Initially patients experience flulike symptoms very similar to EBOLA and MARBURG diseases. Patients may experience eye pain and sensitivity to light and develop a yellow tint to the skin and eyes (jaundice). The less than 1% of patients who develop hemorrhagic fever will bleed from their mucous membranes (eyes, mouth, lining of the nose) and could suffer liver and kidney failure and go into shock. Complications could include inflammation of the brain (encephalitis).

HANTAVIRUS (causing hemorrhagic fever and renal failure): Patients experience sudden onset of intense headache, backache, fever, and chills. Hemorrhage, if it occurs, is manifested as flushed face, petechiae, and bleeding of the eyes (with eye pain) and mucous membranes. As the fever stage ends, low blood pressure can abruptly develop and last for hours to days, during which nausea and vomiting are common. Poor kidney function follows. The final phase can last weeks to months before recovery is complete. Death may occur by kidney failure, respiratory failure, or severely low blood pressure unresponsive to treatment (shock).

YELLOW FEVER: Initially patients experience flulike symptoms very similar to EBOLA and MARBURG. Flushing of the face often occurs. Patients either recover or enter a short remission period followed by fever, slowed heartbeat, yellow tint to the skin and eyes (jaundice), kidney failure, and bleeding complications.

EMERGENCY RESPONSE

- **If you might have been exposed to an airborne release of a VHF virus:**
  - Cover your mouth and nose with fabric (wet if possible) or a respiratory mask.
  - Remove clothes and place in double plastic sealed bags.
  - Wash body thoroughly with soap and water (shower if possible).
  - Thoroughly rinse out your eyes, inside of the nose, lips, and the inside of your mouth. A 0.9% saline eye wash is recommended for flushing out the eyes.
- **Limit contact with infected persons.**

- **Wash immediately and thoroughly with soap and water** any parts of your body (shower if possible) exposed to blood, body fluids, secretions, or excretions from patients with suspected VHF infection.

- **A powered-air purifying respirator (PAPR), or a respiratory mask, and protective clothing (such as gowns and gloves)** must be worn if around patients who are coughing, vomiting, or bleeding, or have diarrhea.

- **Thoroughly decontaminate any object, clothing, or material** an infected person has come in contact with using a 10% bleach solution.

TESTING AND DIAGNOSIS

Clinical microbiology and public-health laboratories are not currently equipped to make a rapid diagnosis of any of these viruses, and blood specimens would need to be sent to the Centers for Disease Control or the U.S. Army Medical Research Institute of Infectious Diseases.

The diagnosis of VHF should be initially based on clinical evidence and judgment, with laboratory testing used to confirm or exclude this clinical diagnosis. Laboratory testing will require time and, in the event of a large attack, may be delayed or perhaps not possible.

TREATMENT

The **antiviral drug ribavirin** is not approved by the Food and Drug Administration for this use, but studies show it may help the symptoms and outcome of some VHFs, such as LASSA, NEW WORLD, and RIFT VALLEY FEVERS. Results have been mixed in its efficacy against HANTAVIRUS, and trials are ongoing. Ideally it should be administered intravenously, but in a mass-casualty setting it can be given in pill form. Treatment should begin once the patient develops symptoms while waiting for culture results to return from the laboratory.

Blood transfusions may be needed in cases of severe bleeding.

Large amounts of **intravenous (IV) fluids** may be necessary, along with medications to maintain blood pressure.

A mechanical breathing device (**ventilator**) may be required in cases of respiratory failure and/or **dialysis** in cases of kidney failure.

Anti-seizure medication may also be required.

Do not use aspirin, as it will diminish the blood-clotting process.

VACCINE

The only viral hemorrhagic fever for which there is a licensed vaccine is YELLOW FEVER. Immune globulin therapy has not been found to be effective.

CHILDREN

- The use of ribavirin for children is not approved by the Federal Drug Administration, and proper doses have not been established. However, if it is one of the more deadly VHFs, the benefits of ribavirin would outweigh the possible risks. Dosages would be reduced from the adult recommendation.
- Ribavirin is not made in capsule dosages for children, and the capsules cannot be broken apart, so a pediatric syrup form is recommended. This syrup is not commercially available and must be obtained by your physician; the maker is Schering-Plough Corporation, in Kenilworth, NJ.

PREGNANCY

- Pregnant women are more likely than others to die from a viral hemorrhagic fever.
- While under normal circumstances ribavirin would not be recommended for pregnant women due to risk to the fetus (as suggested in animal studies), if it is one of the more deadly VHFs, the benefits would outweigh the risks and thus ribavirin may be recommended.

ENVIRONMENTAL DECONTAMINATION AND CLEANUP

Surfaces, equipment, and other articles can be decontaminated by using a 10% bleach solution or a disinfectant like Lysol.

HOW YOU CAN PREPARE

Keep on hand:
- 0.9% saline eye wash
- Respiratory mask
- Insect repellent if mosquito vector is identified

Keep health-facility and emergency phone numbers readily available (see *ADDITIONAL RESOURCES* below and the *Public Resources and Contact Information* section of the book).

ADDITIONAL RESOURCES

American College of Physicians-American Society of Internal Medicine
www.acponline.org/bioterro/hemo_fevers.htm

Centers for Disease Control (CDC)
www.cdc.gov/ncidod/dvrd/spb/mnpages/dispages/vhf.htm

Centers for Disease Control: Chemical/Biological/Radiological Hotline
for obtaining information
Hotline: 888-246-2675

Centers for Disease Control: National Immunization Hotline
Hotline: 800-232-2522

National Institutes of Health
www.nlm.nih.gov/medlineplus/hemorrhagicfevers.html

National Response Center: Chemical/Biological/Radiological Hotline
for reporting incidents
Hotline: 800-424-8802

State public-health locator for officials, agencies, and public hotlines
www.statepublichealth.org

The Survival Guide: What to Do in a Biological, Chemical, or Nuclear
Emergency website: For updates, supplementary information, and
helpful links
www.911guide.com

U.S. Army Medical Research Institute of Infectious Diseases (USAMRIID)
www.usamriid.army.mil
Response Line: 888-USA-RIID (888-872-7443)
Questions or Comments: USAMRIIDweb@amedd.army.mil

VIRAL HEMORRHAGIC FEVERS

DISEASE	Virus Family	Found in Nature	How You Catch It	Person-to-Person Transmission?	Days from Exposure to Illness	DISTINCTIVE SYMPTOMS: In addition to the generalized symptoms, these help identify one VHF from another	Treatment	Possibility of Death
Ebola	Filovirus	Africa	Unknown	Yes	3–16	A spread-out pink rash with solid bumps by day 5 of illness	None	50–90%
Marburg	Filovirus	Africa	Unknown	Yes	3–16	Non-itchy rash with solid bumps on face, neck, torso, and arms may develop	None	23–70%
Lassa Fever	Arenaviridae	Africa	Rodents	Yes	5–16	Gradual onset of fever; flushing of the face and torso, may develop rash and nervous system abnormalities such as tremors and seizures; late stages include severe swelling of face and neck; bleeding complications are less common; may cause deafness	Ribavirin	15–20%
New World Hemorrhagic Fever	Arenaviridae	Americas	Rodents	Yes	7–14	Gradual onset of fever, flushing of face and torso, possible nervous system abnormalities such as tremors of tongue and upper extremities and seizures	Ribavirin	15–30%
Rift Valley Fever	Bunyaviridae	Africa	Mosquitoes, or contact with infected livestock	No	2–5	Eye pain, sensitivity to light, and yellow tint to the skin and eyes (jaundice); less than 1% develop hemorrhagic fever	Ribavirin	Less than 1%
Hantavirus Infection	Bunyaviridae	Asia, Europe, North and South America, possibly worldwide	Rodents		9–35	Hemorrhagic symptoms (flushed face, petechiae) accompany kidney malfunction; life-threatening low blood pressure or pulmonary failure may also occur	Ribavirin (mixed results)	1–15%
Yellow Fever	Flaviviridae	Tropical Africa, South America, Caribbean	Mosquitoes	No	3–6	Flushing of the face; patients either recover or enter a short remission period followed by fever, slowed heartbeat, yellow tint to the skin and eyes (jaundice), kidney failure, and bleeding complications	None	20%

UNIDENTIFIED BIOLOGICAL AGENT

DISEASE
Unidentified

TYPE
Bacteria, virus, or toxin

EARLY POSSIBLE SYMPTOMS

Early symptoms of exposure to a biological agent could include flulike symptoms such as fever, chills, sweats, malaise, fatigue, headache and muscle and joint pain; also nasal and/or lung congestion, breathing difficulties, rash, bumps on skin (solid or pus-filled), weakness, loss of muscle control

EMERGENCY RESPONSE

- Wash hands regularly with soap, particularly after coming in from outside or returning from a public place
- If exposed to an airborne release of an unknown substance and no immediate illness occurs, it may be a biological (versus a chemical) agent:
  - A respiratory mask could be used as a precautionary measure; cover mouth and nose with fabric (wet if possible) if a mask is not available
  - Stay in place for decontamination by emergency personnel if instructed to do so; otherwise, seek shelter
  - Turn off ventilation systems such as air-conditioning (making sure you have enough air to breathe); close all doors, windows, and fireplace dampers
  - Place clothing and items touched in double plastic sealed bags, wash body thoroughly with soap and water (rinse eyes and the inside of the mouth and nose with water), and contact physician or health official
  - Listen to television or radio for emergency announcements
- You may be instructed to "shelter-in-place" for a period of time (see *SPECIAL PRECAUTIONS* section below)
- In the event of an epidemic illness of unknown origin:
  - Keep your distance from infected persons
  - Use respiratory precautions around infected persons and decontaminate contacted clothing and objects with a disinfectant such as a mild bleach solution

TREATMENT

Do **not** begin drug treatment until you have been instructed to do so by an authorized medical professional

VACCINE

If the threat is not completely identified, delay any vaccine until further evidence or confirmation

OVERVIEW

Of all of the biological weapons chapters in this book, this may be one of the most helpful to read, since a situation could occur in which an aerosolized spray of an unknown substance is released or there is a growing epidemic of disease by an initially unidentified bacteria, virus, or toxin. In other words, you might need to act before all of the evidence is in.

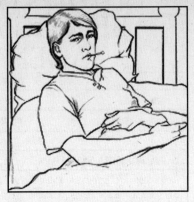

A biological attack may at first go unnoticed and be thought to be a naturally occurring outbreak. Though awareness is currently greatly enhanced, growing numbers of people could fall ill before a deliberate attack was identified by public-health officials.

Many experts believe that a biological attack would not occur in an obvious way, such as from a low-flying crop duster spraying over an open-air football stadium or from powder spewing from an air vent. An event such as this would provoke immediate decontamination and preventive medical tactics that would greatly control a mass outbreak of illness. Therefore, a secret attack may be more likely; an intentionally—possibly suicidal—infected person could start an epidemic by spreading a disease within a crowd; or food, water, or a ventilation system could be imperceptibly contaminated. It is even possible that animals or insects that have contact with humans could be deliberately infected. Because biological agents work by invading the body and generally take hours to days to begin working, an illness could be spread from person to person before we would even know what was happening.

Numerous simulations have been devised to study the course of an intentional infectious outbreak. In 1970 the World Health Organization assessed worst-case scenarios of the dissemination of plague and anthrax, analyzing what would happen if 50 kilograms of either organism were dropped by aircraft release upwind of a city of 5 million. They estimated that around 36,000 (plague) to 100,000 (anthrax) people would die and many more become sick, overwhelming both emergency services and healthcare systems. A 1993 report by the U.S. Congressional Office of Technology Assessment estimated that between 130,000 and 3 million deaths could follow an aerosolized release of 100 kilograms of anthrax spores upwind of the Washington, D.C., area—a lethality similar to that of a hydrogen bomb. While the current climate of awareness and preparedness would likely rein in the extent of these predicted casualties, many factors dictate how one of these scenarios would play out and there is no telling what a real-life outcome would be.

Table 2. Comparison of Biological and Chemical Weapons

Biological Agents	Chemical Agents
Delivered by airborne sprays, weapons, animals, or insects	Delivered by airborne sprays or weapons
Entry primarily through ingestion or inhalation and sometimes through the skin	Entry primarily through inhalation and skin absorption and sometimes by ingestion
Many successfully treated with antibiotics	Treated with antidotes and neutralizing agents
Effects are delayed, usually by days to weeks after exposure	Effects are often immediate or delayed by minutes to a few hours
Agents often not readily available	Components of many agents easy to obtain
Production generally requires scientific knowledge and is expensive	Production can be simple and inexpensive
May be affected by environmental conditions	Affected greatly by environmental conditions

NATIONAL, STATE, AND LOCAL RESPONSES TO AN ATTACK

The Centers for Disease Control (CDC) has very sophisticated means to identify the beginning of an epidemic, particularly one that could be the product of an attack. Since September 11, 2001, the U.S. government has increased the budget of terrorism preparedness and response for state and local health departments through the CDC tenfold. One of the cardinal signs that they look for is a large number of cases of a certain illness over a short period, especially if it is a rare disease and/or from out of the region it naturally occurs in. Most of the biological agents in this book are on watch lists, and cases seen are required by law to be reported to the CDC by those making diagnoses (hospitals, laboratories, and doctors). The CDC has also stepped up its surveillance by monitoring things like records of emergency-room visits, pharmacy purchases, 911 calls, Poison Control Center calls, and the health of the animal population.

The National Pharmaceutical Stockpile, part of the CDC, includes 12 collections that each consist of about 100 huge emergency-response cargo containers, placed strategically at 10 sites around the country. Called "push packs," they are filled with antibiotics, vaccines, antidotes, antitoxins, and other medical supplies that can be delivered anywhere in the United States within 12 hours in the event of an emergency.

Acts of domestic terrorism are under the jurisdiction of the federal government, so several federal agencies become involved to respond to them, starting with the FBI and a criminal investigation. The state health department of incident origin would start its own investigation, and metropolitan health departments and emergency-management teams would also be involved. If an epidemic is threatening to expand beyond a city into the rest of the country and beyond, the World Health Organization (WHO) would probably become involved, and travel notifications would be introduced.

TIMELINE OF ILLNESS

Biological agents can cause illness anywhere from hours to years after exposure; most take several days to a couple of weeks to develop.

INDICATORS OF A POSSIBLE BIOLOGICAL INCIDENT

Table 3.

Unusual numbers of sick or dying people and/or animals	A large number of casualties could indicate that a biological incident has taken place; any number of symptoms could occur—most likely would be gastrointestinal illnesses and upper respiratory problems similar to flu/colds; the time before symptoms are observed depends upon the biological agent and dose received so is highly variable (hours to years)
Unscheduled and unusual aerial spraying	Especially if outdoors during periods of darkness
Abandoned spray devices	Devices would have no distinct odors

(From *"Chemical/Biological/Radiological Incident Handbook,"* by the Chemical, Biological, and Radiological (CBRN) Subcommittee, 1998.)

POSSIBLE EARLY SYMPTOMS

See **Table 4** below.

EMERGENCY RESPONSE

INHALATION:

- **Wash hands regularly with soap,** particularly after coming in from outside or being in a public place. As the majority of infections are spread this way, adopting this habit will prevent everyday infections as well.

- **If you are exposed to an airborne release of an unknown substance and no immediate illness occurs,** it may be a biological (versus a chemical) agent:
  - A respiratory mask could be used as a precautionary measure; if a mask is not available, cover mouth and nose with fabric (wet if possible). Try not to breathe until out of the immediate vicinity; take shallow breaths if you have to breathe.
  - Cover exposed skin.
  - Stay in place for decontamination by emergency personnel if instructed to do so; otherwise, evacuate the area and seek shelter.
  - Place clothing and items touched in double plastic sealed bags, wash body vigorously with germicide soap and water (rinse the eyes and inside of the mouth and nose with water), and contact a physician or health official.
  - Turn off ventilation systems inside your shelter, including fans, air-conditioners, and forced-air heating units. Close doors, windows, and fireplace dampers. If you are instructed to seal your windows, doors, and vents with duct tape, be sure to maintain enough ventilation to prevent suffocation.
  - Listen to television or radio for emergency announcements.
- **You may be instructed to shelter-in-place** for a period of time if public-health officials suspect that a biological agent is still in the air (see *SPECIAL PRECAUTIONS*).
- **If you are evacuating, go against the wind if possible.**
- **In the event of an epidemic illness of unknown origin:**
  - Keep your distance from infected persons.
  - Use respiratory and contact precautions around infected persons and decontaminate contacted clothing and objects with a bleach solution.
- **Call 911 to report an incident.** The National Response Center also has a hotline for reporting biological, chemical, and radiological incidents at 800-424-8802. Give the attendant as much information as you can possibly remember, especially the color and odor of any substance and the condition of any observed victims.

TESTING AND DIAGNOSIS

Healthcare professionals use various clues to distinguish between bioterrorist activity and normal disease. Among these are:
- Severe disease in previously healthy people
- An unusual number of rapidly fatal cases

- A higher than normal number of people with fever, respiratory illnesses including pneumonia, gastrointestinal illnesses, rash, and/or systemic infection
- Disease appearing in an unusual location or time of year
- Multiple people with similar complaints from the same location

Testing and confirmation of samples can take anywhere from a half-hour to several weeks, not counting travel time for getting a specimen to an appropriate, authorized laboratory.

TREATMENT

Do *not* begin drug treatment until you have been instructed to do so by an authorized medical professional. It is extremely important to keep in mind that unnecessary and frequent sporadic use of antibiotics could kill the weakest bacteria and leave the strongest to keep reproducing and causing infection. In this way, we could build antibiotic-resistant bacteria, or bacteria that cannot be killed by common (or possibly any) antibiotics. Furthermore, allergic reactions to antibiotics are not uncommon and can even be life-threatening, and they may also cross-react with other medications you are taking.

The U.S. government has antibiotics, antiviral, and antitoxin treatments stockpiled for our nation in the case of most possible attacks. Once the disease or agent is identified, these will be used.

You may be directed to take medicine or be vaccinated as a preventive measure, even if you are not near an exposure area.

VACCINE

You will be instructed as to whether public-health officials will begin a vaccination (also known as immunization) program. If there is a very high degree of suspicion that an outbreak of a known deadly disease is starting, a vaccination program may begin before absolute laboratory confirmation has been achieved.

There are no vaccinations that are self-administered, so you will need to go to an authorized medical professional to obtain one. Public vaccination centers will be set up by the CDC when they deem it necessary. Vaccination programs are usually initiated with caution, as a small number of people could have serious side effects and even die from getting certain vaccinations.

CHILDREN

- Children are often more susceptible to illnesses caused by biological agents than are adults because their immune systems are not fully

developed yet. In addition, they breathe faster than adults, which could potentially put them at greater risk for inhalational biological agents. Hence, parents should take extra care in decontaminating their children and their surroundings in the event of a suspected exposure to a biological contaminant, to seek medical care, and to monitor them for any signs of developing illness (especially for fever, cough, rash, sluggishness, and difficulty breathing).
- Some of the antibiotics that have special precautions for infants and children are chloramphenicol, ciprofloxacin, doxycycline, streptomycin, tetracycline, trimethoprim-sulfamethoxazole (Bactrim).

PREGNANCY

- Some bacteria and viruses, and the illnesses themselves, could be harmful to a developing fetus. For this reason, pregnant women should take extra care in decontaminating themselves and their surroundings in the event of a suspected exposure to a biological contaminant, to seek medical care, and to monitor themselves for any signs of developing illness (especially fever, cough, and rash).
- Pregnant women should not take any antibiotics unless discussing it first with their doctor.

SPECIAL PRECAUTIONS

Bioengineering: Sophisticated laboratories could possibly engineer bacteria or a virus to be even more deadly than they would be if they occurred naturally, which would usually be done through DNA manipulation. The largest bioterror concern is bacteria that have been made more drug-resistant or contagious or viruses made more virulent. Other ways to make an organism more deadly include special milling to refine particle size (for spores or toxins) to make it more readily aerosolized, and adding agents such as stabilizers to make the organism persist in the environment longer. With such changes, symptoms and/or treatment might be altered as well; hence, it is extremely important to be alert for messages from public-health officials in the event of an outbreak.

In the event of a large biological attack, antibiotics may not be readily available: hospitals, clinics, and pharmacies are not stocked to service entire communities, and supplies would probably be used up immediately. Medications delivered by the National Pharmaceutical Stockpile (of the Centers for Disease Control) could take 12 hours to arrive, or considerably longer if there were distribution difficulties. In addition, if you were asked to "shelter-in-place," you would not be able to get to them.

If you have antibiotics on hand and an unknown infectious disease breaks out:

1) Do *not* begin drug treatment until you have been instructed to do so by an authorized medical professional, and

2) If you have been told to take the antibiotics you have, note the expiration date, as the shelf life for most antibiotics is approximately 2 years.

See the dangers of self-prescribing antibiotics in the *TREATMENT* section above.

You may be asked to **shelter-in-place** for a period of time. If you are outside when the alert is given, try to remove clothing and shoes; place them in a sealed plastic bag and leave them outside before entering your shelter. The safest place in your home would be an inner room without windows. Turn off any ventilation systems and close doors, windows, and fireplace dampers. If you are instructed to seal your windows, doors, and vents with duct tape, be aware that you must maintain enough ventilation to prevent suffocation. Keep water, food with a long shelf life, bedding, medicines, and anything else you may need for at least a 3-day stay in the shelter room (see Chapter 33, *Preparedness and Response Supplies*, for more suggestions on what to store).

ENVIRONMENTAL DECONTAMINATION AND CLEANUP

- For many biological agents, decontaminating potentially exposed surfaces with a 0.5% hypochlorite solution (1 part household bleach added to 9 parts water) would be effective.
- The safest procedure to follow for clothing or other fabric that might be contaminated is to seal them in double plastic bags until told by public-health officials what to do.

HOW YOU CAN PREPARE

10 Tips for Preventing the Spread of Infection

Everyone can help control diseases and prevent infections from spreading by taking certain measures. The Association for Professionals in Infection Control and Epidemiology offers the following ten tips to remember:

1. Wash your hands frequently with soap and water—especially before preparing food, before eating, and after using the restroom (see below). Insist that your healthcare providers wash their hands and use gloves, especially before any invasive treatment or procedure.

2. Don't insist that your physician give you antibiotics if you don't need them. Antibiotics have no effect on illnesses caused by viruses.

3. Take prescribed antibiotics exactly as instructed; do not stop taking them before checking with your physician, even if the medicine makes you feel better—or worse.

4. Keep your immunizations—and those of your children—up to date.
5. Don't send your child to a day care center or school with symptoms of an infection (e.g., vomiting, diarrhea, and/or fever).
6. Follow safe sexual practices.
7. Do not share IV drug needles.
8. Don't share personal items such as razor blades, toothbrushes, combs, and hairbrushes, and don't eat or drink from others' plates or glasses.
9. Keep kitchen surfaces clean, especially when preparing meat, chicken, and fish; disinfect kitchen surfaces.
10. Keep hot foods hot and cold foods cold, especially when they will be left out for a long time.

Hand Washing

Washing hands is such an important means of infection control that it is worth mentioning the most effective technique, as outlined by the College of American Pathologists:

- Use soap and running water.
- Lather well.
- Wash all surfaces, including between your fingers, the backs of your hands, wrists, and under your fingernails.
- Wash thoroughly for 10–15 seconds (ask your children to say their ABCs while they wash to ensure that they spend enough time).
- Rinse well.
- Make it a habit, especially before meals and after using the bathroom, whether you are sick or not.

Note that they do *not* recommend antibacterial or germicide soaps on a regular basis for the same reason that public-health officials do not recommend unnecessary antibiotic use: there is a danger in killing off the weakest bacteria such that only the hardiest survive, thus creating antibacterial-resistant bacteria. Recent studies show that for long-term use ordinary soaps are just as effective. (Germicide soap is recommended for short-term biological agent exposure, however.)

Keep doctor, emergency, and health-facility phone numbers readily available (see *ADDITIONAL RESOURCES* below and the *Public Resources and Contact Information* section of the book). Beginning treatment at the very earliest moment possible would increase your chance of survival for certain fast-moving diseases such as anthrax and pneumonic plague.

Over-the-counter items that may be useful in a biological attack:

Activated charcoal

Eye wash (0.9% saline solution)

Germicide hand and body soap

Insect repellent

Respiratory masks (disposable)

Surface cleaners: disinfectant / germicide / 0.5% bleach solution
(1 part household bleach to 9 parts water)

Duct tape and garbage bags for sealing shelter

ADDITIONAL RESOURCES

Centers for Disease Control (CDC): Chemical/Biological/Radiological
Hotline for obtaining information
www.cdc.gov, www.bt.cdc.gov
Hotline: 888-246-2675

Centers for Disease Control: National Immunization Hotline
www.cdc.gov/nip
Hotline: 800-232-2522

Federal Bureau of Investigation (FBI) Operations Center
www.fbi.gov/terrorinfo/terrorism.htm
Phone: 202-324-6700

Federal Emergency Management Agency (FEMA)
www.fema.gov
Phone: 202-646-4600

Medline-plus Health Information: Medical information from the
National Library of Medicine and the National Institutes of Health
www.nlm.nih.gov/medlineplus/medlineplus.html

National Response Center: Chemical/Biological/Radiological Hotline
for reporting incidents
Hotline: 800-424-8802

State public-health locator for officials, agencies, and public hotlines
www.statepublichealth.org

U.S. Army Medical Research Institute of Infectious Diseases
(USAMRIID)
www.usamriid.army.mil
Response Line: 888-USA-RIID (888-872-7443)
Questions or Comments: USAMRIIDweb@amedd.army.mil

U.S. Food and Drug Administration (FDA)
www.fda.gov/oc/opacom/hottopics/bioterrorism.html

World Health Organization (WHO)
www.who.int/home-page

Table 4. POSSIBLE EARLY SYMPTOMS

	Anthrax (Inhaled)	Botulism (Inhaled)	Brucellosis	Glanders (Inhaled)	Melioidosis (Inh)	Plague (Pneu)	Plague (Bubonic)	Psittacosis	Q Fever	Ricin	Smallpox	T2 Mycotoxin	Tularemia	VHFs*
GENERAL														
Generalized flulike symptoms	X		X	X	X	X	X		X	X	X		X	X
Fever	X		X	X	X	X	X		X	X	X		X	X
Ill feeling (malaise)	X			X	X	X	X		X		X		X	X
Chills	X		X	X	X	X	X		X		X		X	X
Muscle pain	X		X	X	X	X	X		X	X	X		X	X
Joint pain			X						X	X	X			X
Swollen lymph nodes	X (in chest)		X	X	X	Sometimes cervical	X			X (injected)			X	
Weakness			X						X	X		X	X	X
Weight loss			X										X	
Nosebleed												X		X
INTESTINAL														
Stomach pain			X			X	X			X	X	X		X
Diarrhea			X	X	X	X	X		X	X		X		X
Vomiting			X			X	X		X	X	X	X		X
Bloody vomit												X		X
SKIN														
Bumps (solid or pus-filled)			X	X	X						X	X	X	
Ulcers	X			X	X							X	X	
Rash				X	X	X	X		X			X		X
Bruising						X	X							X

POSSIBLE EARLY SYMPTOMS *continued*

	Anthrax (Inhaled)	Botulism (Inhaled)	Brucellosis	Glanders (Inhaled)	Melioidosis (Inh)	Plague (Pneu)	Plague (Bubonic)	Psittacosis	Q Fever	Ricin	Smallpox	T2 Mycotoxin	Tularemia	VHFs*
NEUROLOGICAL														
Muscle weakness / paralysis		X										X		
Confusion / delirium									X		X			X
Blurred or double vision		X										X		
Dizziness		X										X		
Difficulty speaking		X												
Difficulty swallowing		X												
Headache			X	X	X	X	X		X		X		X	X
Eye pain												X	X	
RESPIRATORY														
Chest pain	X		X	X	X	X			X			X	X	
Cough	X		X			X			X	X	X	X	X	
Congestion (lung and nasal)	X^L			X	X	X^L			X^L	X^L		X	X	
Breathing difficulties	X	X				X			X	X		X	X	
Bloody phlegm						X						X		X

* Viral hemorrhagic fevers (VHFs) include Ebola, Marburg, hantavirus, and Lassa, Rift Valley, and yellow fevers. L = Lung only.

AGENT 15

CHEMICAL AGENT	TYPE
Agent 15	Psychoactive agent

CHARACTERISTICS

Can exist as an odorless solid, liquid, or gas

HOW YOU GET EXPOSED

Can be inhaled, ingested, or absorbed through the skin

TIME FROM EXPOSURE TO ILLNESS

30 minutes to 36 hours

MAJOR SYMPTOMS

Dilated (enlarged) pupils, blurred vision, dry mouth, dry skin, illusions, hallucinations, denial of illness, impaired memory, and short attention span

EMERGENCY RESPONSE

- Leave the vicinity of attack immediately and seek fresh air
- Cover mouth and nose (with a wet cloth if possible), and try not to breathe until away from the area
- If exposed, remove clothing and shower with soap and water
- Gas masks or air-purifying respirators are required for emergency responders working at the scene; however, the use of gas masks by the untrained is not recommended due to the danger of improper use

TREATMENT

The antidote physostigmine

POSSIBILITY OF DEATH

Effects are nonlethal and temporary

ANTIDOTE

Exists

WHAT IT IS

Agent 15 is a chemical known as a "psychotomimetic" agent because its effects often mimic psychotic disorders. The effects are transient and primarily cause incapacitation due to hallucinations and irrational behavior.

It is alleged that Iraq developed large stocks of Agent 15 as a gas. It appears to be very similar to another agent called BZ, which was weaponized by the United States at one time (it was deweaponized in 1988).

Agent 15 could be dispersed as an aerosol or dissolved in liquid to allow for ingestion or skin absorption. It could also be converted into a gas.

WHAT IT DOES

Following absorption via inhalation, ingestion, and/or skin, Agent 15 alters the communication between nerves. Initially this causes blood vessels to dilate, which causes the skin to warm and redden without perspiration or the ability to dissipate heat. Body temperature rises as a result. As it gets into the brain, Agent 15 affects the nerve junctions there and alters mental processes.

HOW DO YOU TELL WHAT IT IS?

Since pure Agent 15 would be odorless and nonirritating, the primary way to recognize it would be to note the symptoms in yourself and those around you. These symptoms may begin with blurred vision, dry mouth, and short attention span. One aspect of Agent 15's effects is that a victim would deny that anything is wrong with herself—hence, if these symptoms begin in a potential attack area, it is essential to leave the vicinity at once.

Some of the prominent symptoms are the opposite of what you would see in a nerve agent attack: dilated (enlarged) pupils and dry mouth. With a nerve agent, pupils would shrink and salivation would be overstimulated to the point of drooling.

ASSESSMENT OF RISK

Risk of Use in an Attack

Compounds similar to Agent 15 in their effects are present in plants such as jimsonweed, black henbane, belladonna, and Jerusalem cherry, making it potentially easy to obtain components to make it or something like it. Only a tiny amount (e.g., 100 mg) would be sufficient in aerosolized form to incapacitate.

How Dangerous Is It?

Its effects are nonlethal and temporary. The greatest danger to victims' lives is from (1) injuries due to their own erratic behavior and (2) high body temperature. A severely exposed patient may go into a coma with acute heartbeat irregularities and electrolyte disturbances.

TIMELINE OF ILLNESS

Symptoms appear 30 minutes to 24 hours after exposure, and up to 36 hours later for skin exposure. There are 4 stages of symptom development after exposure:

Stage	Time Period	Symptoms
I	0–4 hours	Mostly mild, peripheral central-nervous-system effects such as dry mouth, dilated pupils, and flushed, red, warm skin
II	4–20 hours	Stupor, lack of coordination, increased body temperature
III	20–96 hours	Delirium, which fluctuates from moment to moment
IV	Resolution	Paranoia, deep sleep, and crawling or climbing impulses, with eventual reorientation. Symptoms usually last 72–96 hours but effects can remain for 1–3 weeks

SYMPTOMS

Characteristic symptoms of Agent 15 poisoning are dilated (enlarged) pupils, blurred vision, dry mouth, dry skin, illusions, hallucinations, denial of illness, impaired memory, and short attention span.

The skin becomes warm from decreased sweating and red from dilated blood vessels. Secretions are generally decreased—so that mouth, eyes, nose, and throat are dry; gastrointestinally, constipation results. Heart rate increases at first, then slows down. Consciousness decreases, beginning with drowsiness and possibly progressing to stupor and coma. Disorientation, disturbances in judgment and inappropriate behavior, slurred speech, and monotonous voice might also be evident. Another characteristic finding is behavioral changes ranging from quiet confusion to combativeness followed by paranoia. When groups of people are affected, the group shares hallucinations (mass hysteria) and is highly prone to suggestion: for example, people could take turns smoking an imaginary cigarette—visible to them but no one else!

EMERGENCY RESPONSE

- **Leave the vicinity of attack immediately and seek fresh air.** Cover your mouth and nose (with a wet cloth if possible), and try not to breathe until away from the area. Take shallow breaths if you need to breathe.

- **If exposed, remove clothing and shower with soap and water.** Place clothes in two plastic, sealed bags. Trained professionals will handle further decontamination.

- **There is no need to protect oneself from people already exposed,** as the agent is absorbed rapidly into the system.

- **Gas masks or air-purifying respirators** are required for emergency responders working at the scene; however, the use of gas masks by the untrained is not recommended due to the danger of improper use.

- **Specialized protective clothing** is necessary for emergency responders working at the scene to prevent the agent from being absorbed into the skin.

TESTING AND DIAGNOSIS

No environmental detector is available that could be of immediate clinical use. Confirmation of release is made by laboratory analysis of environmental specimens, but this requires a great deal of time on the part of trained professionals. Doctors may be able to make the diagnosis much more quickly based on clinical signs and symptoms.

TREATMENT

The **antidote** (see below) can be administered, or patients can be given mild sedatives until their symptoms resolve.

ANTIDOTE

There is very little data on Agent 15, but U.S. Army guides suggest that BZ and Agent 15 are essentially very similar; hence, antidote recommendations are based on BZ. The antidote, **physostigmine**, is minimally effective in the early hours of exposure (up to 4 hours) but is subsequently very effective. Physostigmine does not shorten the course of poisoning, so relapses will occur if treatment is prematurely discontinued.

CHILDREN

The dose of the antidote (physostigmine) must be adjusted for children.

PREGNANCY

No special precautions.

SPECIAL PRECAUTIONS

Since one feature of Agent 15 poisoning is that the victim would not be aware that he is intoxicated and could exhibit irrational, erratic behavior, it would be important to keep close watch on an exposed person so he would not harm himself.

ENVIRONMENTAL DECONTAMINATION AND CLEANUP

The U.S. Army Medical Research Institute of Chemical Defense manual states that Agent 15 would be extremely persistent in soil and water and on many surfaces. It is particularly stable in moist conditions and could remain active for many weeks.

HOW YOU CAN PREPARE

Keep health-facility and emergency phone numbers readily available (see *ADDITIONAL RESOURCES* below and the *Public Resources and Contact Information* section of the book).

Note that a charcoal-activated gas mask, while protective, would likely be impractical in the event of an attack. It weighs about 4 pounds, and you would have to carry it everywhere to be ready for a surprise strike. If you choose to purchase one for your home, you must read the instructions carefully and practice with it, as improper use will not protect you and could actually suffocate you. WARNING: Our medical experts do not recommend the use of gas masks except by trained professionals. Data from Israel shows that the incorrect use of gas masks has caused many fatalities.

ADDITIONAL RESOURCES

Centers for Disease Control: Chemical/Biological/Radiological Hotline
    for obtaining information
      Hotline: 888-246-2675
National Response Center: Chemical/Biological/Radiological Hotline
    for reporting incidents
      Hotline: 800-424-8802
State-public health locator for officials, agencies, and public hotlines
    www.statepublichealth.org

The Survival Guide: What to Do in a Biological, Chemical, or Nuclear
  Emergency website: For updates, supplementary information, and
  helpful links
  www.911guide.com
The U.S. Army Medical Research Institute of Chemical Defense
  (USAMRICD)
  chemdef.apgea.army.mil
  Phone: 410-436-3628
  3100 Ricketts Point Road
  Aberdeen Proving Ground, MD 21010-5400

BLISTER AGENTS: Lewisite

CHEMICAL AGENT	TYPE
Lewisite	Blister agent (vesicant)

CHARACTERISTICS

Oily, colorless liquid at room temperature; can be odorless or smell like geraniums

HOW YOU GET EXPOSED

Primarily inhalation and absorption through the skin and mucous membranes (especially the eyes)

TIME FROM EXPOSURE TO ILLNESS

Vapor or liquid causes immediate pain or irritation (unlike mustard gas)

MAJOR SYMPTOMS

Immediate burning of skin, large blister formation, eye and airway irritation, violent sneezing, sore throat, cough, chest pain, profuse mucus in nasal passages and airways, fluid-filled lungs, possible nausea and vomiting

EMERGENCY RESPONSE

- Leave the area of exposure at once; seconds count
- Cover your nose and mouth with cloth (wet if possible)
- Try not to inhale until you are out of the area of exposure; if you must breathe, take shallow breaths
- Unless it inhibits your escape, try to close your eyes, as blister agents can cause permanent eye damage and blindness within minutes
- Blister agents are heavier than air. Do *not* go below ground level, do *not* lie on the floor or ground
- If exposed, remove clothing and rinse skin with copious amounts of water (shower if possible), even if symptom-free: severity of skin injury depends upon how quickly the skin is decontaminated.
- Flush eyes with water for 10–15 minutes
- Seek medical attention immediately: skin antidote should be administered as soon as possible
- Gas masks or air-purifying respirators are required for emergency responders working at the scene; however, the use of gas masks by the untrained is not recommended due to the danger of improper use

TREATMENT

Antidote; large blisters (1–2 cm) drained and cleansed; topical antibiotics for skin infections and/or systemic antibiotics for bacterial pneumonia and acquired skin infections; iodophors such as Betadine for skin; for eye care, petroleum jelly and anticholinergic eye solutions

POSSIBILITY OF DEATH

Usually low (2–3%) but could be higher with concentrated exposure

ANTIDOTE

Exists

WHAT IT IS

Lewisite (military code name L) is a blister agent—also known as a "vesicant"—that painfully burns and blisters the skin or any other part of the body it contacts. It is a liquid at room temperature and vaporizes to form a gas, both forms of which are hazardous; on hot, humid

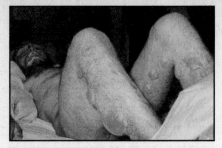

Man showing the large blistering effects of a blister agent.

days it is even more harmful to human tissue. Generally fast-acting, all chemical reactions relating to tissue injury are complete within minutes. It can enter the body through many routes: breathing in, ingestion, and absorption through the skin and eyes. In addition to penetrating the cells of tissues, lewisite can penetrate a great number of materials as well, such as wood, leather, and rubber.

Lewisite was first isolated in pure form in the United States by W. L. Lewis in 1918. It was developed as an alternative, less persistent agent than mustard gas, which would make it easier to stage attacks across a contaminated battleground. When lewisite was being shipped to Europe, World War I ended, so it was destroyed at sea and never used. Armed forces are interested in it because of its effectiveness as an incapacitator, since troops would be blinded and blistered if unprotected, or at the very least would become less mobile, having to wear bulky, full-body equipment to protect themselves.

Blister agents are considered second only to nerve agents as a concern to the U.S. military.

WHAT IT DOES

Lewisite inhibits vital DNA function and kills off the most rapidly dividing cells first (skin cells and the lining of the stomach).

It causes blistering of the skin and mucous membranes. The tissue of eyes, respiratory tract, and genitalia are particularly susceptible to blister burns. Warm, moist areas of the body are most vulnerable, such as the groin, the crease of the forearm, and the neck.

Death is usually due to respiratory failure, secondary bacterial pneumonia, and mechanical obstruction by sloughing mucous membranes within the airways, causing the inability to move air in and out of the lungs. Death can also occur with severe spasm of the larynx (voice box), causing the victim to choke.

AEROSOL: Lewisite damages the respiratory tract when inhaled. It easily penetrates clothing and blisters the skin; large burns may lead to life-threatening lung injury. The intestines are also damaged. Systemic poisoning can lead to hemoconcentration (loss of fluids in the vascular system), low blood pressure, shock, and death.

INGESTED: Ingestion of contaminated food or water may cause destruction of the gastrointestinal tract lining.

CONTACT: The eyes are most susceptible and would be affected at even very low concentrations.

HOW DO YOU TELL WHAT IT IS?

It should be noted that the following descriptions are not hard and fast rules because lewisite may be mixed with other chemicals or substances that would change its physical characteristics:

LEWISITE: The pure compound is a colorless, odorless, oily liquid. Industrially produced lewisite is amber to dark brown and has a strong geranium odor. Exposure induces immediate, burning pain.

MUSTARD GAS (another blister agent) may be combined with LEWISITE: This combination would probably smell like garlic.

ASSESSMENT OF RISK

Risk of Use in an Attack
Lewisite is of great concern because it can be easily manufactured and is quickly incapacitating as well as deadly.

How Dangerous Is It?
Lewisite is more volatile than mustard gas, which makes it harder to maintain a potent vapor concentration, and it also causes more severe burns. Mortality is usually low (2–3%), but it could be higher with concentrated exposure.

TIMELINE OF ILLNESS

Lewisite causes a rapid onset of symptoms. Stinging pain is usually felt within 10–20 seconds after contact with the liquid. Within a few minutes the pain becomes deep and aching. After 5 minutes, a gray area of dead skin appears, resembling an acid burn. Itching and irritation persists for about 24 hours, whether or not blisters develop. If blisters do appear, they are often well developed by 12 hours and are very painful at first. After 48–72 hours the pain lessens. Breathing in this agent will cause immediate, severe injury to the respiratory tract.

EYES: Eye irritation begins immediately. Mild cases of eye exposure will recover in 1–2 weeks. More severe damage may take 2–5 weeks for recovery. When the corneas are damaged, permanent scarring may occur; recovery may take 2–3 months. Severe corneal involvement may cause temporary blindness, though permanent blindness is rare.

SKIN: Skin is damaged within 5 minutes and blister formation is complete in 12–18 hours. Surface lesions heal in 14–21 days. Deep blisters can take up to 60 days to heal.

RESPIRATORY TRACT: Earliest symptoms include respiratory and eye complaints, although it is difficult to define a time course. Some patients show persistent damage.

Early: sore throat, cough, hoarseness
12–14 hours: shortness of breath
3-4 days: bacterial lung infections (pneumonia) with increased phlegm production and fever
5–10 days: death, though rare, may occur due to infection and respiratory failure

POSSIBLE LONG-TERM EFFECTS: Visual impairment (permanent blindness is rare), scarring of the skin, chronic bronchitis, bronchial stenosis (narrowing of the airways), and increased sensitivity to blister agents. In addition, blister agents are cancer-causing compounds: World Wars I and II mustard-gas victims showed an increased incidence of lung cancer.

LEWISITE/MUSTARD GAS combination: Delayed onset.

SYMPTOMS

INHALED/INGESTED: There is immediate burning in the chest. Early symptoms (seconds to minutes after exposure) are hoarseness, sore throat, cough, and chest pressure, as well as profuse nasal secretions and violent sneezing. There may be spasms of the windpipe and breathing obstruction due to mucus and dead tissue plugging the airways. Fluid may develop in the lungs (edema). Nausea and vomiting could also occur.

SKIN: Immediate stinging pain. Skin redness develops within 30 minutes, with pain and itching for 24 hours. Depending on the concentration of exposure, large blisters may form on the skin within 12 hours, lasting 2–3 days. The blisters may or may not be painful, but the lesions left behind after they rupture would likely be quite painful. Vapor exposure to skin could cause deep burns (first- to second-degree); liquid exposure may result in burn penetration to the full thickness of the skin. Symptoms of inhalation may also accompany skin effects (see above). High environmental temperature and wet skin are associated with more severe and rapid onset of symptoms. Skin lesions change from red to brownish-purple to black over time. Wounds tend to heal slowly, taking from several weeks to several months. Scarring may occur. With lewisite, wounds are deeper and more tissue death occurs than with mustard gas.

EYES: Pain, irritation, pain when looking at bright light, blurred vision, and swelling of the eyelids. Inflammation and scarring of the cornea. Severe permanent damage or blindness is rare.

SYSTEMIC: Absorption through any route, including severe skin exposure, may cause headache, abdominal pain, nausea, and vomiting. Absorption of high doses could cause convulsions and heartbeat irregularities that could lead to a heart attack. Acute systemic poisoning from large skin burns (larger than the palm of the hand or covering more than 5% of the body) leads to lung injury (symptoms of this are cough with shortness of breath and frothy saliva possibly tinged with blood). Other symptoms are diarrhea, restlessness, weakness, and low blood pressure. This is a very serious, life-threatening condition.

EMERGENCY RESPONSE

- **Vacate the vicinity of the attack at once.**
- **Do not breathe fumes.** If possible, hold your breath—or cover your mouth with whatever wet fabric you can find—until out of the exposure area or until a respiratory mask is in place. A positive-pressure, full-face, self-contained breathing apparatus is the best defense. A gas mask with activated charcoal filters is next best. These respiratory masks are recommended only for emergency responders trained in their use; we do not recommend the purchase or use of them by the untrained.
- **Unless it inhibits your escape, try to keep your eyes closed** if possible during a gas attack, as permanent damage to the eyes, including blindness, can occur within minutes. Due to severe swelling of eyelids and the lining of the eye, the eyes may swell shut within 1 hour.
- **Avoid skin contact with the agent at all times.**
- **Remove clothes, and shower with copious amounts of water** if you think you have been exposed, even if you are symptom-free. If decontamination is not done immediately, injury to the skin cannot be prevented (later decontamination can only limit the severity of damage).
- **A 0.5% bleach solution (1 part bleach, 9 parts water) has been shown to inactivate these compounds,** but since copious amounts of water are effective for decontamination, time should not be wasted attempting to formulate bleach solutions. Never put bleach in the eyes.

- **Flush eyes with water for 10–15 minutes** as soon as you are able to.
- **Lewisite is heavier than air:** Do *not* go below ground level; do *not* lie on the floor or ground.
- **Seek medical attention *immediately*** if exposed.
- **The skin antidote dimercaprol** should be administered as soon as possible.

TESTING AND DIAGNOSIS

Lewisite can be detected by observing color change in certain liquid mixtures. There is no automatic environmental detector. There is no specific diagnostic test for humans to confirm lewisite exposure.

TREATMENT

Begin **antidotes** as soon as possible (see *ANTIDOTE* section below).

SKIN: As the skin turns red and itches intensely, application of **cooling preparations** (e.g., calamine lotion or water) will help ease this effect. Ointments and creams are not advised. Blisters greater than 2 cm should be drained and an **antibiotic cream** such as Bacitracin applied. Once the blisters have broken, it is best to remove the "roof" of dead skin and irrigate with a saline solution 4 times per day to reduce the possibility of infection. For very large blisters, patients may require whirlpool-bath **irrigation**. Infection of wounds is a serious complication for blister-agent patients, thus appropriate intravenous antibacterial preparations should be used. **Pain-relief medication** may be necessary.

Recent research suggests that **iodophors** such as povodine iodine (Betadine) may limit skin toxicity. Since these agents are relatively benign and available, bathing or washing in povodine would be encouraged immediately following exposure. Caution: It is not to be used in the eyes.

EYES: **Petroleum jelly** may be applied to the edges of the eyelids and **anticholinergic solutions** in the eyes. **Topical antibiotics** are applied several times a day.

RESPIRATORY: The airway must be opened and secured to allow for the suctioning of lung secretions. **Oxygen** would likely need to be administered as soon as possible. A **ventilator** (breathing machine) may be necessary for severe breathing difficulties. Mild symptoms such as hoarseness and sore throat do not usually need to be treated. Cough may be relieved by codeine. If bacterial pneumonia develops (usually 3–4 days post-exposure), intravenous antibiotics must be administered. **Broncho-dilators** and **steroids** may be needed for airway spasms.

ANTIDOTE

The effects of lewisite can be prevented by the rapid application to the skin of **dimercaprol** (2,3-dimercaptopropanol, also known as British Anti-Lewisite, or BAL), which reacts with lewisite to form a nontoxic product. If possible, any protective ointment already on the skin should be removed first. Dimercaprol eye ointment may diminish the effects on the eyes if applied within 2 minutes of exposure; its value after this is questionable. While dimercaprol is an effective antidote, it is in very short supply and not readily available.

CHILDREN

No special precautions.

PREGNANCY

Blister agents are teratogenic, meaning they can cause severe developmental abnormalities to an embryo or fetus. Thus, medical counseling post-exposure is strongly recommended for the pregnant woman.

SPECIAL PRECAUTIONS

As it only takes seconds to become affected by lewisite, leaving your shelter to rescue or assist victims during an ongoing release could be a deadly decision. Bear in mind that there is likely little help the untrained could offer that would be of any value to a victim of this chemical agent.

People who are contaminated with certain chemical agents may pose a danger to those who give them mouth-to-mouth resuscitation. It is difficult to determine this risk in an emergency situation when the particular agent or concentration of the exposure is unknown. As a precaution, a pocket resuscitation mask could be purchased; this is a curved plastic cup that rests over the victim's mouth and has a short tube attached for the rescuer to blow into. Note that if a patient appears wet, it may be residual liquid blister agent.

ENVIRONMENTAL DECONTAMINATION AND CLEANUP

- Blister agents can be thickened into an oily liquid that can remain on surfaces as a persistent hazard.
- Lewisite is stable below about 120°F and is not inactivated by exposure to sunlight.
- Blister agents are very persistent in cold and temperate climates. In warmer weather, they are less persistent, though concentrations of vapor would be higher and more potent.

– The primary mode for decontamination of blister agents is copious amounts of water with a 0.5% hypochlorite bleach solution (1 part bleach, 9 parts water). Protective respiratory support and clothing must be worn by trained personnel.

HOW YOU CAN PREPARE

Ordinary clothing provides little protection from blister agents—they can even pass through rubber. Specialized protective equipment would need to be used, including a respirator, a specialized suit, gloves, and overboots, which should be used by trained emergency responders and professionals.

Note that a charcoal-activated gas mask, while protective, would likely be impractical in the event of an attack. It weighs about 4 pounds, and you would have to carry it everywhere to be ready for a surprise strike. If you choose to purchase one for your home, you must read the instructions carefully and practice with it, as improper use will not protect you and could actually suffocate you. WARNING: Our medical experts do not recommend the use of gas masks except by trained professionals. Data from Israel shows that the incorrect use of gas masks has caused many fatalities.

ADDITIONAL RESOURCES

Agency for Toxic Substances and Disease Registry (ATSDR)
  www.atsdr.cdc.gov
Centers for Disease Control (CDC)
  www.state.sd.us/doh/bioterrorism/chemical%20agents.pdf
Centers for Disease Control: Chemical/Biological/Radiological Hotline
  for obtaining information: 888-246-2675
Centers for Disease Control (CDC): Lewisite fact sheet
  www.bt.cdc.gov/agent/blister/ctc0020.asp
Federation of American Scientists
  www.fas.org/nuke/intro/cw/agent.htm
National Response Center: Chemical/Biological/Radiological Hotline
  for reporting incidents: 800-424-8802
State public-health locator for officials, agencies, and public hotlines
  www.statepublichealth.org
The Survival Guide: What to Do in a Biological, Chemical, or Nuclear
  Emergency website: For updates, supplementary information, and
  helpful links
  www.911guide.com
U.S. Army Medical Research Institute of Chemical Defense
  (USAMRICD)
  ccc.apgea.army.mil
  Phone: 410-436-2230

BLISTER AGENTS: Mustard Gas

CHEMICAL AGENT	TYPE
Mustard Gas	Blister agent (vesicant)

CHARACTERISTICS

Oily liquid at room temperature; color is yellow to brown; smells like garlic, onion, or mustard, or can be nearly odorless

HOW YOU GET EXPOSED

Primarily inhalation and absorption through the skin and mucous membranes (especially the eyes)

TIME FROM EXPOSURE TO ILLNESS

Damage to tissue may occur in minutes, but the onset of symptoms due to the underlying tissue damage may not occur for 2–48 hours; heavy exposure may cause mild skin and eye symptoms in under an hour

MAJOR SYMPTOMS

Red, itching, and/or burning skin; large blister formation; eye and airway irritation; violent sneezing, sore throat; cough; chest pain; profuse mucus in nasal passages and airways; possible nausea and vomiting

EMERGENCY RESPONSE

- Leave the area of exposure at once; seconds count
- Cover your nose and mouth with cloth (wet if possible)
- Try not to inhale until you are out of the area of exposure; if you must breathe, take shallow breaths
- Unless it inhibits your escape, try to close your eyes, as blister agents can cause permanent eye damage and blindness within minutes
- Blister agents are heavier than air: Do *not* go below ground level, do *not* lie on the floor or ground
- If exposed, remove clothing and rinse skin with copious amounts of water (shower if possible), even if symptom-free: severity of skin injury depends on how quickly the skin is decontaminated
- Flush eyes with water for 10–15 minutes
- Seek medical attention immediately: skin treatment should be administered as soon as possible
- Gas masks or air-purifying respirators are required for emergency responders working at the scene; however, the use of gas masks by the untrained is not recommended due to the danger of improper use

TREATMENT

Paste containing chlorinating agent or iodophors for skin detoxification; large blisters (1–2 cm) must be drained and cleansed; topical antibiotics for skin infections and/or systemic antibiotics for bacterial pneumonia and acquired skin infections; for eye care, petroleum jelly and anticholinergic eye solutions

POSSIBILITY OF DEATH

Usually low (2–3%) but could be high with strong concentration of exposure

ANTIDOTE

None exists

WHAT IT IS

Mustard gas (military code names HD, HN, and HT) is a blister agent, also known as a "vesicant," that painfully burns and blisters the skin or any other part of the body it contacts. It is a liquid at room temperature and vaporizes to form a gas, both forms of which are hazardous; on hot, humid days it is even more harmful to human tissue. Generally fast-acting, all chemical reactions

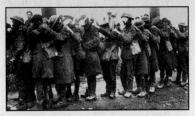

Soldiers seeking medical treatment at a dressing station after returning from the battlefield where mustard gas was used near the end of World War I. About 1.3 million gas-related casualties, including over 91,000 deaths, occurred during World War I.

relating to tissue injury are complete within minutes. It can enter the body through many routes: breathing in, ingestion, and absorption through the skin and eyes. In addition to penetrating the cells of tissues, mustard gas can penetrate a great number of materials as well, such as wood, leather, and rubber.

Mustard gas has been used in warfare since the early 1900s. It was used in both world wars. It was also used by Egypt against Yemen in the 1960s and in the Iran-Iraq war of the 1980s. Armed forces use it because of its effectiveness as an incapacitator, since troops would be blinded and blistered if unprotected, or at the very least would be required to wear bulky, full-body equipment to protect themselves from it, making them less effective in battle. Mustard gas and other blister agents are considered second only to nerve agents as a concern to the U.S. military.

WHAT IT DOES

Mustard gas inhibits vital DNA function and kills off the most rapidly dividing cells first (such as skin cells, the lining of the stomach, and all elements of the bone marrow). It causes blistering of the skin and mucous membranes. Tissues of the eyes, respiratory tract, and genitalia are particularly susceptible to blister burns. Warm, moist areas of the body are most vulnerable, such as the groin, crease of the forearm, and neck. Death is usually due to respiratory failure, bone marrow suppression, secondary bacterial pneumonia, and mechanical obstruction by sloughing mucous membranes within the airways, causing the inability to move air in and out of the lungs. Death can also occur with severe spasm of the larynx (voice box), causing the victim to choke.

AEROSOL: Mustard gas damages the respiratory tract when inhaled. It easily penetrates clothing and blisters the skin; large burns may lead to life-threatening lung injury. The intestines are also damaged. Systemic poisoning can lead to hemoconcentration (loss of fluids in the vascular system), low blood pressure, shock, and death.

INGESTED: Ingestion of contaminated food or water may cause destruction of the gastrointestinal-tract lining.

CONTACT: The eyes are most susceptible and would be affected at even very low concentrations.

HOW DO YOU TELL WHAT IT IS?

It should be noted that the following descriptions are not hard-and-fast rules because mustard gas may be mixed with other chemicals or substances that would change its physical characteristics:

MUSTARD GAS: Depending on the type, mustard gas can range from a colorless to pale yellow to dark brown oily liquid (at room temperature). It can smell like garlic, onion, or mustard, or it can be odorless to some people. It may taste like garlic. There is no pain at the time of exposure. Its effects appear hours after exposure.

LEWISITE (another blister agent) may be combined with MUSTARD GAS: This combination would probably smell like garlic.

ASSESSMENT OF RISK

Risk of Use in an Attack
Mustard gas is of great concern because it can be easily manufactured and is incapacitating as well as deadly.

How Dangerous Is It?
Historically, mustard gas is the most feared of the blister agents due to its stability and persistence in the environment and because of its insidious effects of attacking skin as well as eyes and the respiratory tract, with no effective counteractive therapy. Mortality is usually low (2–3%), but it could be greater with concentrated exposure.

TIMELINE OF ILLNESS

Although a drop of mustard agent on the skin can cause serious damage within 2 minutes, the onset of symptoms as a result of the tissue damage may be delayed by hours to days. For this reason, it is important that anyone who might have been exposed in an attack is thoroughly decontaminated whether they are expressing symptoms or not.

EYES: Symptoms may not set in for several hours. Mild cases of eye exposure will recover in 1–2 weeks; more severe damage may take 2–5 weeks. When the corneas are damaged, permanent scarring may occur;

recovery may take 2–3 months. Severe corneal involvement may cause temporary blindness, though permanent blindness is rare.

SKIN: Concentrated exposure may cause reddening of skin within 30 minutes to an hour. There could be a period of 2–48 (usually 4–12) hours after exposure with no symptoms, then skin could redden (erythema), progressing to blister formation and skin death. Surface lesions heal in 14–21 days. Deep blisters can take up to 60 days to heal.

RESPIRATORY TRACT: Earliest symptoms are respiratory, although it is difficult to define a time course. Some patients show persistent damage.

Early:	Sore throat, cough, hoarseness
12–14 hours:	Shortness of breath
3–4 days:	Bacterial lung infections (pneumonia) with increased phlegm production and fever
5–10 days:	Death, though rare, may occur due to infection and respiratory failure

POSSIBLE LONG-TERM EFFECTS: Visual impairment (permanent blindness is rare), scarring of the skin, chronic bronchitis, bronchial stenosis (narrowing of the airways), and increased sensitivity to blister agents. In addition, blister agents are cancer-causing compounds: World Wars I and II mustard-gas victims showed an increased incidence of lung cancer.

MUSTARD/LEWISITE combination: Delayed onset.

SYMPTOMS

INHALED/INGESTED: There is no immediate pain. Early symptoms (minutes to hours after exposure) are hoarseness, sore throat, cough, and chest pressure. There may be profuse nasal secretions and violent sneezing. Spasms of the windpipe and breathing obstruction may occur due to mucus and dead tissue plugging the airways. Fluid may develop in the lungs (edema). Destruction of mucous membranes and nausea and vomiting could also occur.

SKIN: No immediate pain. Skin redness may occur within 30 minutes, and pain and itching may follow in the next 24 hours. Depending on the concentration of exposure, large blisters may form on the skin within 12 hours; blistering can go on for several days before reaching its maximum and last 2–3 days. After that, crops of new blisters may appear as late as the second week after exposure. The blisters may or may not be painful, but they are fragile and the lesions left behind after they rupture would likely be quite painful. Vapor exposure to skin could cause deep burns (first- to second-degree); liquid exposure may result in burn penetration to the full thickness of the skin. Symptoms of inhalation may also accompany skin effects (see above). High environmental temperature and wet skin are associated with more severe and rapid onset of symptoms. Skin lesions change from red to brownish-purple to black over time. Wounds tend to heal slowly, taking from several weeks to several months. Scarring may occur.

EYES: After a symptom-free period of around 1–12 hours, a victim may experience a sensation of grit in the eyes. Other symptoms are pain, irritation, pain when looking at bright light, blurred vision, and swelling of the eyelids, along with inflammation and scarring of the cornea. Severe permanent damage or blindness is rare.

SYSTEMIC: Absorption through any route, including severe skin exposure, may cause headache, abdominal pain, nausea, and vomiting. Absorption of high doses could cause convulsions and heartbeat irregularities that could lead to a heart attack. Acute systemic poisoning from large skin burns (larger than the palm of the hand or covering more than 5% of the body) leads to lung injury (symptoms of this are cough with shortness of breath and frothy saliva possibly tinged with blood). Other symptoms are diarrhea, restlessness, weakness, and low blood pressure. This is a very serious, life-threatening condition.

EMERGENCY RESPONSE

- **Vacate the vicinity of the attack at once.**
- **Do not breathe fumes.** If possible, hold your breath—or cover your mouth with whatever wet fabric you can find—until out of the exposure area or until a respiratory mask is in place. A positive-pressure, full-face, self-contained breathing apparatus is the best defense. A gas mask with activated charcoal filters is next best. These masks are recommended only for emergency responders trained in their use; we do not recommend the purchase or use of them by the untrained.
- **Unless it inhibits your escape, try to keep your eyes closed** during a gas attack, as permanent damage to the eyes, including blindness, can occur within minutes. Due to severe swelling of eyelids and the lining of the eye, the eyes may swell shut within 1 hour.
- **Avoid skin contact with the agent at all times.**
- **Remove clothes, and shower with copious amounts of water** if you think you have been exposed, even if you are symptom-free. If decontamination is not done immediately, injury to the skin cannot be prevented (later decontamination can only limit the severity of damage).
- **A 0.5% bleach solution (1 part bleach, 9 parts water) has been shown to inactivate these compounds,** but since copious amounts of water are effective for decontamination, time should not be wasted attempting to formulate bleach solutions. Never put bleach in the eyes.

- **Flush eyes with water for 10–15 minutes** as soon as you can.
- **Mustard gas is heavier than air:** Do *not* go below ground level; do *not* lie on the floor or ground.
- **Seek medical attention *immediately*** if exposed.
- **Skin treatment** should be administered as soon as possible.

TESTING AND DIAGNOSIS

Mustard gas can be detected in the environment by a number of means. Special colorized detector paper is available to the military. Monitoring devices for local contamination and water-testing kits are also available. Clinically, the gas and its metabolite (thiodiglycol) can be detected in urine for up to a week.

TREATMENT

There is no drug available for the effects of mustard gas on the skin and mucous membranes. Recent research suggests that **iodophors** such as povodine iodine (Betadine) may limit skin toxicity. Since these agents are relatively benign and available in every hospital and pharmacy without a prescription, washing in povodine would be encouraged immediately following exposure. Caution: these are also not to be used in the eyes.

SKIN: As skin turns red and itches intensely, application of **cooling preparations** (e.g., calamine lotion or water) will help ease this effect. Ointments and creams are not advised. Blisters larger than 2 cm should be drained and an **antibiotic cream** such as Bacitracin applied. Once the blisters have broken, it is best to remove the "roof" of dead skin and irrigate with a saline solution 4 times per day to decrease the possibility of infection. For very large blisters, patients may require whirlpool-bath **irrigation**. Infection of wounds is a serious complication for blister-agent patients, thus appropriate intravenous antibacterial preparations should be used. **Pain-relief medication** may be necessary.

EYES: **Petroleum jelly** may be applied to the edges of the eyelids and **anticholinergic solutions** in the eyes. **Topical antibiotics** are applied several times a day.

RESPIRATORY: The airway must be opened and secured to allow for the suctioning of lung secretions. **Oxygen** would likely need to be administered as soon as possible. A **ventilator** (breathing machine) may be necessary for severe breathing difficulties. Mild symptoms such as hoarseness and sore throat do not usually need to be treated. Cough may be relieved by codeine. If bacterial pneumonia develops (usually 3–4 days post-exposure), intravenous antibiotics must be administered.

Bronchodilators and **steroids** may be needed for airway spasms.

ANTIDOTE

No specific antidote exists.

CHILDREN

The time to the onset of symptoms may be shorter and severity of skin injury greater in children compared to adults. In addition, eye, lung, and gastrointestinal lesions are more common in children than adults.

PREGNANCY

Blister agents are teratogenic, meaning they can cause severe developmental abnormalities to an embryo or fetus. Thus, there is great need for medical counseling post-exposure for the pregnant woman.

SPECIAL PRECAUTIONS

As it only takes seconds to become affected by mustard gas, leaving your shelter to rescue or assist victims during an ongoing release could be a deadly decision. Bear in mind that there is likely little help the untrained could offer that would be of any value to a victim of this chemical agent.

People who are contaminated with certain chemical agents may pose a danger to those who give them mouth-to-mouth resuscitation. It is difficult to determine this risk in an emergency situation when the particular agent or concentration of the exposure is unknown. As a precaution, a pocket resuscitation mask could be purchased; this is a curved plastic cup that rests over the victim's mouth and has a short tube attached for the rescuer to blow into. Note that if a patient appears wet, it may be residual liquid blister agent.

ENVIRONMENTAL DECONTAMINATION AND CLEANUP

- Blister agents can be thickened into an oily liquid that can remain on surfaces as a persistent hazard.
- If mustard gas were released, it would remain in the air or on the ground for about a day. Once in the soil, it could remain active for several weeks without decontamination methods.
- Blister agents are very persistent in cold and temperate climates. In warmer weather, they are less persistent, though higher concentrations of vapor would occur.
- The primary mode for decontamination of blister agents is copious amounts of water with a 0.5% hypochlorite bleach solution (1 part

bleach, 9 parts water). Protective respiratory support and clothing must be worn by trained personnel.

HOW YOU CAN PREPARE

Ordinary clothing provides little protection from blister agents—they can even pass through rubber. Specialized protective equipment would need to be used, including a respirator, a hazardous materials suit, gloves, and overboots, which should be used by trained emergency responders and professionals.

Skin can be protected from very low doses by covering it with a paste containing a chlorinating agent (e.g., chloramines)—note this is for the skin, not for eyes or mucous membranes—though it is neither practical nor readily available.

Note that a charcoal-activated gas mask, while protective, would likely be impractical in the event of an attack. It weighs about 4 pounds, and you would have to carry it everywhere to be ready for a surprise strike. If you choose to purchase one for your home, you must read the instructions carefully and practice with it, as improper use will not protect you and could actually suffocate you. WARNING: Our medical experts do not recommend the use of gas masks except by trained professionals. Data from Israel shows that the incorrect use of gas masks has caused many fatalities.

ADDITIONAL RESOURCES

Agency for Toxic Substances and Disease Registry (ATSDR)
    www.atsdr.cdc.gov
Centers for Disease Control (CDC)
    www.state.sd.us/doh/Bioterrorism/chemical%20agents.pdf
Centers for Disease Control: Chemical/Biological/Radiological Hotline
    for obtaining information: 888-246-2675
Federation of American Scientists
    www.fas.org/nuke/intro/cw/agent.htm
National Response Center: Chemical/Biological/Radiological Hotline
    for reporting incidents: 800-424-8802
State public-health locator for officials, agencies, and public hotlines
    www.statepublichealth.org
U.S. Army Medical Research Institute of Chemical Defense (USAMRICD)
    ccc.apgea.army.mil, Phone: 410-436-2230
U.S. Army Soldier and Biological Chemical Command
    www.sbccom.army.mil/services/edu/mustard.htm

BLISTER AGENTS: Phosgene Oxime

CHEMICAL AGENT	TYPE
Phosgene Oxime	Urticant (causes hives)

CHARACTERISTICS

White, crystalline powder or could be liquefied with added solvents; smell has peppery, unpleasant, pungent odor

HOW YOU GET EXPOSED

Inhalation, ingestion, and absorption through the skin and mucous membranes (especially the eyes)

TIME FROM EXPOSURE TO ILLNESS

Immediate tissue injury

MAJOR SYMPTOMS

Immediate burning of the skin followed by blanching and a red ring around point of contact in 30 seconds, hives in 30 minutes, and skin death later on; extreme pain of skin and eyes may persist for days; airway irritation, sore throat, cough, chest pain, profuse mucus in nasal passages and airways; possibly nausea, vomiting, and bleeding in the gastrointestinal tract

EMERGENCY RESPONSE

- Leave the area of exposure at once; seconds count
- Cover your nose and mouth with cloth (wet if possible)
- Try not to inhale until out of exposure area; if you must breathe, take shallow breaths
- Unless it inhibits your escape, try to close your eyes if possible, as blister agents can cause permanent eye damage and blindness within minutes
- Blister agents are heavier than air: Do *not* go below ground level; do *not* lie on the floor or ground
- If exposed, remove clothing and shower immediately, or rinse skin with lots of water, even if symptom-free: severity of skin injury depends upon how quickly the skin is decontaminated.
- Seek medical attention immediately; skin treatment should be administered as soon as possible
- Flush eyes with water for 10–15 minutes
- Gas masks or purified air respirators are required for emergency responders working at the scene; however, the use of gas masks by the untrained is not recommended due to the danger of improper use

TREATMENT

Iodophors such as Betadine for skin; topical antibiotics for skin infections, and/or systemic antibiotics for bacterial pneumonia and acquired skin infections; for eye care, petroleum jelly and anticholinergic eye solutions

POSSIBILITY OF DEATH

Usually low (2–3%) but could be high with strong concentration of exposure

ANTIDOTE

None exists

WHAT IT IS

Phosgene oxime (military code name CX), although commonly grouped with blister agents, does not cause blisters. It is an "urticant" (causes hives) or "nettle agent" that causes corrosion of tissues. Both the vapor and liquid forms cause immediate, extreme irritation of the skin, mucous membranes, and airways. As a solid, phosgene oxime can decompose spontaneously and must therefore be stored at low temperatures. On hot, humid days it is even more harmful to human tissue. Generally fast-acting, it can enter the body through many routes: inhalation, ingestion, and absorption through the skin and eyes. All chemical reactions relating to tissue injury are complete within minutes, as with blister agents lewisite and mustard gas. In addition to penetrating the cells of tissues, phosgene oxime can penetrate the rubber of protective boots and gloves over time.

WHAT THEY DO

Phosgene oxime has never been used in warfare and there is not much data regarding its effects on humans.

Phosgene oxime inhibits vital DNA function and kills off the most rapidly dividing cells first (skin cells and the lining of the stomach). It causes corrosion of the skin and mucous membranes. The tissues of the eyes, respiratory tract, and genitalia are particularly susceptible to these burns. Warm, moist areas of the body are most vulnerable, such as the groin, crease of the forearm, and neck.

Death is usually due to respiratory failure, secondary bacterial pneumonia, acute lung injury (fluid-filled lungs), and mechanical obstruction by sloughing mucous membranes plugging the airways, causing the inability to move air in and out of the lungs. Death can also occur with severe spasm of the larynx (voice box), causing the victim to choke.

AEROSOL: Phosgene oxime damages the respiratory tract when inhaled. It easily penetrates clothing and burns the skin; large burns may lead to life-threatening lung injury. The intestines are also damaged, and gastrointestinal bleeding can occur. Systemic poisoning can lead to hemo-concentration (loss of fluids in the vascular system), low blood pressure, shock, and death.

INGESTED: Ingestion of contaminated food or water may cause destruction of the gastrointestinal-tract lining.

CONTACT: The eyes are most susceptible and would be affected at even very low concentrations. Compared with blister agents mustard gas and lewisite, phosgene oxime is the most irritating to skin and eyes.

HOW DO YOU TELL WHAT IT IS?

Phosgene oxime is a white, crystalline powder or at room temperature it could be liquefied with added solvents. It may smell like pepper. It causes welts (like hives) on the skin but not blisters. It should be noted that these descriptions are not hard-and-fast rules because phosgene oxime may be mixed with other chemicals or substances that would change its physical characteristics.

ASSESSMENT OF RISK

Risk of Use in an Attack

Phosgene oxime is of concern because it can be easily manufactured and is incapacitating as well as deadly in high concentrations.

How Dangerous Is It?

Phosgene oxime has never been used in battle, so little is known about its effects on humans. Mortality would probably be low (2–3%), but it could be higher with high concentration exposure.

TIMELINE OF ILLNESS

EYES: Extreme eye pain may begin immediately and persist for days. Mild cases of eye exposure will recover in 1–2 weeks. More severe damage may take 2–5 weeks for recovery. When the corneas are damaged, permanent scarring may occur; recovery may take 2–3 months. Severe corneal involvement may cause temporary blindness, though permanent blindness is rare.

SKIN: Extreme skin pain may begin immediately and persist for days. Burning of the skin is followed by blanching and then red ring formation around the point of contact in 30 seconds. Hives follow in about 30 minutes, with skin death later on.

RESPIRATORY TRACT: Earliest symptoms involve the respiratory tract as well as eyes and skin, although it is difficult to define a time course. Some patients may show persistent damage.

Early:	Sore throat, cough, hoarseness
12–14 hours:	Shortness of breath
3–4 days:	Bacterial lung infections (pneumonia) with increased phlegm production and fever
5–10 days:	Death, though rare, may occur due to infection and respiratory failure

Recovery may take 1–3 months. Possible long-term effects include visual impairment (permanent blindness is rare), scarring of the skin, chronic bronchitis, bronchial stenosis (narrowing of the airways), and increased sensitivity to blister agents.

SYMPTOMS

INHALED/INGESTED: There is immediate burning in the chest. Early symptoms (seconds to minutes after exposure) are hoarseness, sore throat, cough, and chest pressure, as well as profuse nasal secretions and violent sneezing. There may be spasms of the windpipe and breathing obstruction due to mucus and dead tissue plugging the airways. Fluid may develop in the lungs. Nausea and vomiting could also occur, as well as gastrointestinal bleeding.

SKIN: Immediate stinging pain. There is burning of the skin, causing welts (like hives) on the skin but not blisters. Redness develops within 30 minutes, with pain and itching for 24 hours. Vapor exposure to skin could cause deep burns (first- to second-degree); liquid exposure may result in burn penetration to the full thickness of the skin. Symptoms of inhalation may also accompany skin effects (see above). High environmental temperature and wet skin are associated with more severe and rapid onset of symptoms. Skin lesions change from red to brownish-purple to black over time. Wounds tend to heal slowly, taking from several weeks to several months. Scarring may occur.

EYES: Pain, irritation, pain when looking at bright light, blurred vision, and swelling of the eyelids. Inflammation and scarring of the cornea. Severe permanent damage or blindness is rare.

SYSTEMIC: Absorption by any route, including severe skin exposure, may cause headache, abdominal pain, nausea, and vomiting. Absorption of high doses could cause convulsions and heartbeat irregularities that could lead to a heart attack. Acute systemic poisoning from large skin burns (larger than the palm of the hand or covering more than 5% of the body) leads to lung injury and pulmonary edema (symptoms of this are cough with shortness of breath and frothy saliva possibly tinged with blood). Other symptoms are diarrhea, restlessness, weakness, and low blood pressure. This is a very serious, life-threatening condition.

EMERGENCY RESPONSE

- **Vacate the vicinity of the attack at once.**
- **Do not breathe fumes.** If possible, hold your breath—or cover your mouth with whatever wet fabric you can find—until out of the exposure area or until a respiratory mask is in place. A positive-pressure, full-face, self-contained breathing apparatus is the best defense. A gas mask with activated charcoal filters is next best. These masks are recommended only for emergency responders trained in their use; we do not recommend the purchase or use of them to the untrained.

- **Unless it inhibits your escape, try to keep your eyes closed** during a gas attack, as permanent damage to the eyes, including blindness, can occur within minutes. Due to severe swelling of eyelids and the lining of the eye, the eyes may swell shut within 1 hour.

- **Avoid skin contact with the agent at all times.**

- **Remove clothes, and shower with copious amounts of water** if you think you have been exposed, even if you are symptom-free. If decontamination is not done immediately, injury to the skin cannot be prevented (later decontamination can only limit the severity of damage).

- **A 0.5% bleach solution (1 part bleach, 9 parts water) has been shown to inactivate these compounds,** but since copious amounts of water are effective for decontamination, time should not be wasted attempting to formulate bleach solutions. Never put bleach in the eyes.

- **Flush eyes with water for 10–15 minutes** as soon as you can.

- **Phosgene oxime is heavier than air:** Do *not* go below ground level; do *not* lie on the floor or ground.

- **Seek medical attention *immediately*** if exposed.

- **Skin treatment** should be administered as soon as possible.

TESTING AND DIAGNOSIS

No automatic environmental detector exists for phosgene oxime. There are also no distinctive laboratory findings for the diagnosis of phosgene oxime exposure in people.

TREATMENT

SKIN: As skin turns red and itches intensely, application of **cooling preparations** (e.g., calamine lotion or water) will help ease this effect. Ointments and creams are not advised. An antibiotic cream such as Bacitracin should be applied to burns. For very large burns, patients may require whirlpool bath irrigation. Infection of wounds is a serious complication for blister agent patients, thus appropriate systemic **antibacterial preparations** should be used. Pain relief medication may be necessary.

Recent research suggests that **iodophors** such as povodine iodine (Betadine) may limit skin toxicity. Since these agents are relatively benign and available, bathing or washing in povodine would be encouraged *immediately* following exposure. Caution: It is not to be used in the eyes.

EYES: Eyes should be flushed with water. **Petroleum jelly** may be applied to the edges of the eyelids and **anticholinergic solutions** in the eyes. **Topical antibiotics** are applied several times a day.

RESPIRATORY: The airway must be opened and secured to allow for the suctioning of lung secretions. **Oxygen** would likely need to be administered as soon as possible. A **ventilator** (breathing machine) may be necessary for severe breathing difficulties. Mild symptoms such as hoarseness and sore throat do not usually need to be treated. Cough may be relieved by codeine. If bacterial pneumonia develops (usually 3–4 days post-exposure), intravenous antibiotics must be administered. **Broncho-dilators** and **steroids** may be needed for spasm of the airway.

ANTIDOTE

No specific antidote exists.

CHILDREN

No special precautions.

PREGNANCY

Blister agents are teratogenic, meaning they can cause severe developmental abnormalities to an embryo or fetus. Thus, medical counseling post-exposure is strongly recommended for the pregnant woman.

SPECIAL PRECAUTIONS

As it only takes seconds to become affected by phosgene oxime, leaving shelter to rescue or assist victims during an ongoing release could be a deadly decision. Bear in mind that there is likely no help the untrained could offer that would be of any value to a victim of a chemical agent.

People who are contaminated with certain chemical agents may pose a danger to those who give them mouth-to-mouth resuscitation. It is difficult to determine this risk in an emergency situation when the particular agent or concentration of the exposure is unknown. As a precautionary measure, a pocket resuscitation mask could be purchased, which is a curved, plastic cup that rests over the victim's mouth and has a short tube attached to blow into for the rescuer. Note that if a patient appears wet, it may be residual liquid blister agent.

ENVIRONMENTAL DECONTAMINATION AND CLEANUP

- Chemical inactivation using alkali is effective. Protective respiratory support and clothing must be worn by the trained professionals who will perform environmental cleanup.
- Blister agents can be thickened into an oily liquid that could remain on surfaces as a persistent hazard.

– Blister agents are very persistent in cold and temperate climates. In warmer weather, they are less persistent, though concentrations of vapor are higher and more potent.

HOW YOU CAN PREPARE

Keep health-facility and emergency phone numbers readily available (see *ADDITIONAL RESOURCES* below and the *Public Resources and Contact Information* section of the book).

Ordinary clothing provides little protection from blister agents —they can even pass through rubber. Specialized protective equipment would need to be used, including a respirator, a hazardous materials suit, gloves, and overboots, which should be used by trained emergency responders and professionals.

Note that a charcoal-activated gas mask, while protective, would likely be impractical in the event of an attack. It weighs about 4 pounds, and you would have to carry it everywhere to be ready for a surprise strike. If you choose to purchase one for your home, you must read the instructions carefully and practice with it, as improper use will not protect you and could actually suffocate you. WARNING: Our medical experts do not recommend the use of gas masks except by trained professionals. Data from Israel shows that the incorrect use of gas masks has caused many fatalities.

ADDITIONAL RESOURCES

Agency for Toxic Substances and Disease Registry (ATSDR)
www.atsdr.cdc.gov
Centers for Disease Control (CDC)
www.state.sd.us/doh/bioterrorism/chemical%20agents.pdf
Centers for Disease Control (CDC): Chemical/Biological/Radiological
Hotline for obtaining information
Hotline: 888-246-2675
Federation of American Scientists
www.fas.org/nuke/intro/cw/agent.htm
National Response Center: Chemical/Biological/Radiological Hotline
for reporting incidents
Hotline: 800-424-8802
State public-health locator for officials, agencies, and public hotlines
www.statepublichealth.org
The Survival Guide: What to Do in a Biological, Chemical, or Nuclear
Emergency website: For updates, supplementary information, and
helpful links
www.911guide.com

U.S. Army Medical Research Institute of Chemical Defense (USAMRICD)
ccc.apgea.army.mil
Phone: 410-436-2230

CHEMICAL ASPHYXIANTS

CHEMICAL AGENTS	TYPE
Arsine, Hydrogen Cyanide, Cyanogen Chloride	Chemical asphyxiant (also known as "blood agents")

CHARACTERISTICS

Usually colorless gases, they can smell like bitter almonds (HYDROGEN CYANIDE, CYANOGEN CHLORIDE) or garlic (ARSINE)

HOW YOU GET EXPOSED

Absorbed by breathing in their vapors and (less so) through the skin and eyes; in some cases, such as in solid compounds or powder, they could also be ingested

TIME FROM EXPOSURE TO ILLNESS

Most are very rapid—death can occur within a few minutes; ARSINE effects may be delayed for up to several hours

MAJOR SYMPTOMS

HYDROGEN CYANIDE
MILD EXPOSURE: Mild irritation to eyes, nose, and airways; shortness of breath, agitation, weakness, nausea, vomiting, muscular trembling; can gradually advance to symptoms of concentrated exposure if not treated
CONCENTRATED EXPOSURE: Same as above with increasing severity, plus sudden increase in deep breaths, vertigo, violent convulsions; can progress rapidly to cessation of respiration and heart failure
CYANOGEN CHLORIDE
Same as above but with greater irritation to eyes, nose, throat, and airways
ARSINE
Early symptoms include red staining of the eyes, garlic breath odor, headache, thirst, shivering, weakness, jaundice, and abdominal pain; severe exposure can lead to kidney failure

EMERGENCY RESPONSE

- Leave the area of exposure at once
- Cover your nose and mouth with fabric (wet if possible)
- Try not to breathe in until you are out of the area of exposure; if you must breathe, take shallow breaths
- Charcoal-activated gas masks are required for emergency responders working at the scene; however, the use of gas masks by the untrained is not recommended due to the danger of improper use
- Seek medical attention immediately; antidote should be administered as soon as possible

TREATMENT

Antidote kit (except ARSINE); oxygen supplementation; fluid and cardiac support

POSSIBILITY OF DEATH

Can be rapidly fatal, depending on concentration of exposure

ANTIDOTE

Antidote treatment kit exists for CYANIDE poisoning; no antidote for ARSINE

WHAT THEY ARE

Chemical asphyxiants (also known as "blood agents") are rapidly acting, lethal chemicals that are absorbed into the body primarily by breathing in their vapors; they can also be absorbed in lesser amounts through the skin and eyes. The chemicals are generally stored as liquids, but once a container is opened and

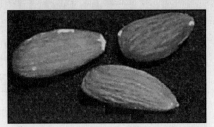

Some chemical asphyxiants, such as hydrogen cyanide and cyanogen chloride, may have the smell of bitter almonds.

they are exposed to the air, they rapidly become gases and expand to a wide area. Chemical asphyxiants interfere with oxygen utilization; once they spread through the bloodstream and enter cells, they cause death by suffocation.

CYANIDE (military code name CN) is of the most concern for use as a potential chemical weapon and exists in different forms: HYDROGEN CYANIDE (AC) (also called HYDROCYANIC ACID [HCN]) and CYANOGEN CHLORIDE (CK). ARSINE (SA) will also be discussed in this chapter.

Chemical asphyxiants have been used in warfare since the time of Napoleon III. The French used about 4,000 tons of cyanide in World War I without notable military success due to its high volatility (it is unstable and evaporates immediately), its quick dispersion, and the high concentration needed. In a confined area these gases would be much more dangerous, since they would be present in higher concentrations and thus require much less to be lethal.

WHAT THEY DO

Normally red blood cells transport oxygen to tissues of the body and deliver it to cells. Cyanide prevents tissue uptake of oxygen. This mechanical breakdown, leaving oxygen in the circulation, often causes the blood to become bright red and gives the skin a red, flushed cast in the early stages.

ARSINE destroys red blood cells altogether as well, so there are fewer blood cells left to deliver oxygen throughout the body. In addition to depriving the body of oxygen, arsine also causes kidney and liver damage.

HOW DO YOU TELL WHAT IT IS?

The presence of a chemical asphyxiant would primarily be detected by the symptoms you and others around you were experiencing. They are usually only mildly irritating to the eyes, nose, and throat (in contrast to the corrosive, burning sensation of pulmonary irritants), but they could rapidly cause breathing difficulties and respiratory failure, possibly within minutes. The following includes general qualities for pure gases—it should be noted that these are not hard-and-fast indicators because the gases could be mixed with other chemicals or substances that would change their characteristics.

HYDROGEN CYANIDE: A colorless gas or liquid, hydrogen cyanide can smell like bitter almonds. Only 60–80% of the population can detect the bitter almond odor of cyanide, with 3 times more women being able to smell it than men.

CYANOGEN CHLORIDE: Cyanogen chloride is a colorless gas that can smell weakly of bitter almonds. It also causes a burning sensation in the eyes, throat, and lungs.

ARSINE: Arsine is a colorless gas that smells mildly of garlic. Effects could be delayed for up to several hours rather than be immediate. Arsine is sometimes mixed with the nerve agent lewisite to cause an immediate irritant and skin-damaging effect.

ASSESSMENT OF RISK

Risk of Use in an Attack

Because CYANIDES are used in industry, their availability is one reason that terrorists might choose to use them. They can also be found in very small quantities in the fruits and seeds (especially pits) of many plants, such as cherries, peaches, almonds, and lima beans, as well as in certain bacteria, fungi, and algae. However, the volatile properties of chemical asphyxiants make them less desirable since they dissipate so quickly—for example, ARSINE is so volatile that it can explode on contact with the air.

How Dangerous Is It?

CYANIDE gases would be very dangerous in an unventilated, enclosed space; however, in the open air massive amounts would be needed to create a deadly concentration. Death may occur quickly following exposure to an extremely concentrated gas. With oral exposure, symptoms may be somewhat delayed but can be equally as lethal.

ARSINE is highly toxic at extremely low concentrations; death may occur quickly following an extremely concentrated exposure.

TIMELINE OF ILLNESS

HYDROGEN CYANIDE: Onset of symptoms is very rapid. After inhalation of high concentration, hyperventilation may occur for approximately 15 seconds, followed within 15–30 seconds by convulsions. Breathing stops 2–3 minutes later, and heart stops several minutes after that (approximately 6–8 minutes after exposure).

CYANOGEN CHLORIDE: Onset of symptoms is rapid.

ARSINE: Onset of symptoms is usually 30–60 minutes after exposure, but effects may be delayed for up to several hours. In a high enough concentration, death could occur rapidly.

SYMPTOMS

HYDROGEN CYANIDE

Initial Symptoms: Mild irritation to eyes, nose, and airways, flushing of the skin, rapid heartbeat, rapid breathing, headache, dizziness, high blood pressure.

Mild/Moderate Symptoms: Nausea, vomiting, palpitations, agitation, anxiety, vertigo, confusion, hyperventilation, weakness, muscular trembling.

Severe Symptoms: Same as above with increasing severity, plus sudden increase in deep breaths, inability to hold breath, absence of breathing, slowed heartbeat, low blood pressure, irregular heartbeat, fluid-filled lungs (acute lung injury), a dark blue or purplish coloration to the skin due to the lack of oxygen (late stage), stupor, coma, respiratory and heart failure.

CYANOGEN CHLORIDE

Same as above but with greater irritation to eyes, nose, throat, and airways.

ARSINE

Symptoms may appear as early as 30–60 minutes after exposure, or patients may look and feel well for several hours before symptoms set in.

Early Symptoms: Red eyes, garlic breath odor, headache, thirst, and shivering.

Later Symptoms: Abdominal pain, jaundice (yellow tint to the skin), generalized weakness, muscle cramps, and occasionally low blood pressure. Loss of appetite, nausea, and vomiting sometimes occur. Urine may be red or dark brown.

Late-Stage Symptoms: Jaundice, and kidney impairment possibly leading to kidney failure in severe cases.

EMERGENCY RESPONSE

- **Leave the area of exposure immediately** and seek fresh air. If you can, try not to breathe in before you are away from the vapors. If you must breathe, take shallow breaths.
- **Cover your nose and mouth with fabric** (wet if possible).
- **Gas masks with activated charcoal filters** are required for emergency responders working at the scene and would need to be changed every 10

minutes. However, the purchase of gas masks is not recommended for the lay person due to the danger of improper use.

- **Antidote treatment** (see below) should be started immediately for patients with symptoms after high-concentration exposure.

- **If exposed, seek medical attention immediately.**

- Because CYANOGEN CHLORIDE is heavier than air, if it is confirmed that this is the gas used, do not go below ground level or lie on the floor or ground. *In contrast,* HYDROGEN CYANIDE and ARSINE are lighter than air, so would rise. Trained emergency personnel will advise you what to do.

TESTING AND DIAGNOSIS

Automatic environmental detectors that can distinguish concentrations of cyanide vapor are available to the military; water testing kits exist as well.

Blood tests in humans would indicate (1) elevated cyanide level, (2) high concentration of lactic acid, and (3) increased content of oxygen in the veins (due to the inability of blood to transfer oxygen into cells). Treatment needs to be given based on clinical signs and symptoms since these tests take a long time for confirmation.

For ARSINE, measurement of blood arsenic levels may be useful. Treatment needs to be given based on clinical signs and symptoms since these tests take a long time for confirmation.

TREATMENT

CYANIDE
INHALED:
- **100% oxygen** supplementation should be started as soon as possible.
- Begin **antidote therapy** (see below) immediately for patients with symptoms of concentrated exposure.
- Victims may need **breathing, circulatory, and cardiac support** using fluids, a breathing machine (ventilator), medication for systemic acidosis, and Valium for seizure control.

INGESTED:
- Induced vomiting and pumping the stomach are of limited value since absorption into the bloodstream is so rapid. **Activated charcoal** should be used despite the low binding of cyanide to the charcoal.

Note: Those who are fully conscious and breathing normally 5 minutes after exposure do not need any treatment because cyanide is very rapidly detoxified in the body.

ARSINE

Similar **breathing and fluid support** as for cyanide poisoning. However, the cyanide antidote kit is ineffective. **Bronchodilators** may be administered for windpipe spasms. **Blood transfusion** and/or **dialysis** may be necessary.

ANTIDOTE

The CYANIDE-poisoning antidote kit consists of the following medications: **amyl nitrite**, **sodium nitrite**, and **sodium thiosulfate**. Amyl nitrite is administered as an ampule (small glass bulb filled with medicine) when intravenous sodium nitrite is not immediately available—it is broken and inhaled for 30 seconds each minute, a new one every 3 minutes. Sodium thiosulfate should be given intravenously immediately following sodium nitrite treatment. Sodium nitrite and thiosulfate therapy can be repeated in half doses 30 minutes later if there is inadequate progress in the patient's condition. These are to be administered by trained professionals.

Some patients may recover without antidote if vigorous supportive therapy is given. Antidote therapy is not without its own risks: if not given slowly enough or in large doses, it can be hazardous.

CHILDREN

For sodium nitrite treatment, dosages *must* be properly adjusted for children, as an incorrect dose can cause a fatal blood condition called methemoglobinemia.

PREGNANCY

No special precautions.

SPECIAL PRECAUTIONS

Exposure to a chemical asphyxiant could be fatal in a matter of minutes. Leaving shelter to rescue or assist victims during an ongoing release could be a deadly decision. Bear in mind that there is likely no help the untrained could offer that would be of any value to a victim of this chemical agent.

ENVIRONMENTAL DECONTAMINATION AND CLEANUP

- Cyanide compounds are slowly inactivated in water.
- Because of their rapid evaporation into the environment, decontamination should not be necessary for most chemical asphyxiants.

- If decontamination is required, protective clothing must be worn by trained professionals. Although the predominant entry for chemical asphyxiants is inhalation, they can also be absorbed through the skin and eyes.

HOW YOU CAN PREPARE

Keep health-facility and emergency phone numbers readily available (see *ADDITIONAL RESOURCES* below and the *Public Resources and Contact Information* section of the book).

While a gas mask with a supply of charcoal-activated filters would protect the eyes and airways from blood-agent fumes, one would have to have immediate access to one. Further, in order to ensure effective use, you must practice beforehand; improper fit could mean the difference between life and death. Note that since filters would need to be changed every 10 minutes, an ample supply of them would be needed. WARNING: Our medical experts do not recommend the use of gas masks except by trained professionals. Data from Israel shows that the incorrect use of gas masks has caused many fatalities.

ADDITIONAL RESOURCES

Centers for Disease Control (CDC)
> *www.state.sd.us/doh/bioterrorism/chemical%20agents.pdf*

Centers for Disease Control: Chemical/Biological/Radiological Hotline
for obtaining information
Hotline: 888-246-2675

National Response Center: Chemical/Biological/Radiological Hotline
for reporting incidents
Hotline: 800-424-8802

State public-health locator for officials, agencies, and public hotlines
www.statepublichealth.org

The Survival Guide: What to Do in a Biological, Chemical, or Nuclear
Emergency website: For updates, supplementary information, and
helpful links
www.911guide.com

U.S. Army Medical Research Institute of Chemical Defense (USAMRICD)
ccc.apgea.army.mil
Phone: 410-436-2230

NERVE AGENTS

CHEMICAL AGENTS	TYPE
Sarin, Soman, Tabun, VX, GF	Nerve gas

CHARACTERISTICS

Most come in the form of colorless and tasteless liquids (golden-brown VX is one exception). They can be odorless or have a slightly fruity, sweet, musty, nutty, or camphor smell

HOW YOU GET EXPOSED

Inhaled, ingested, and in high concentrations absorbed through skin and eyes

TIME FROM EXPOSURE TO ILLNESS

Symptoms begin within seconds to minutes

MAJOR SYMPTOMS

MILD INHALED EXPOSURE: Runny nose, watery eyes, shortness of breath, sweating, sneezing, sudden excess saliva, dimmed or blurred vision
CONCENTRATED EXPOSURE: All of the above symptoms with increased severity; plus drooling, eye pain, involuntary urination and/or defecation, vomiting; red, irritated eyes and nose, blood-tinged saliva and nasal secretions; sudden loss of consciousness, seizures, and paralysis could occur

EMERGENCY RESPONSE

- Leave the area of exposure at once; seconds count
- Cover your nose and mouth with cloth (wet if possible)
- Try not to breathe in until out of exposure area; if you must breathe, take shallow breaths
- Nerve agents are heavier than air: Do *not* go below ground level, do *not* lie on the floor or ground
- If exposed, remove clothing and shower immediately
- Flush eyes with water for 10–15 minutes
- Try to remain calm—it will benefit breathing ability
- Survival depends upon how quickly treatment is started and respiratory support given
- Gas masks or air-purifying respirators are required for emergency responders working at the scene; however, the use of gas masks by the untrained is not recommended due to the danger of improper use

TREATMENT

The antidotes atropine and pralidoxime should begin as soon as possible; Valium can be used for convulsions

POSSIBILITY OF DEATH

Death could occur in 1–10 minutes, depending on concentration of exposure

ANTIDOTE

Available to emergency personnel, medical professionals, and the military

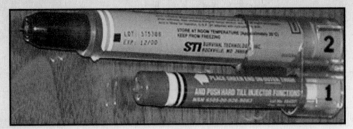

Nerve Agent Antidote Kits (NAAK), also known as Mark-1 kits, would be used in the event of exposure to a nerve agent. The two antidotes, pralidoxime and atropine, are administered to counter the effects of the nerve agent. Currently, these kits are carried by the military and many emergency personnel.

WHAT THEY ARE

Nerve agents are man-made, deadly poisons that attack the nervous system. They are effective because they are generally fast-acting and can enter the body through many routes: inhalation, ingestion, and, in very high concentrations, absorption through the skin and eyes. Many are used in military weapons programs because they are so highly toxic yet break down within days in the environment to become harmless. They are made of chemicals known as organic phosphorous compounds (commonly referred to as "organophosphates"), which are also present in industrial-strength pesticides used in the farming and pharmaceutical industries.

The nerve agents that will be discussed in this chapter (with their military code names in parentheses) are: SARIN (GB), SOMAN (GD), TABUN (GA), and VX. The nerve gas GF, similar to the others in symptoms and treatment, is also included, though less is known about this particular agent.

Nerve agents can be used in three ways as chemical-warfare agents:

1) In a container at normal room temperature, nerve agents are usually liquids and are vaporized when the container is opened; the gas evaporates slowly into the air and would be inhaled. Many nerve gases can be vaporized at room temperature (72°F) or above or if sprayed in an explosion. (Vaporization from packages containing liquid sarin was the method used by a Japanese cult in the Tokyo subway system in 1995, which killed 12 people and injured over 5,000.)

2) They can also be thickened (such as to the consistency of a lubricating oil) so that they do not evaporate quickly but would rapidly absorb into the skin if touched. VX usually comes in this form.

3) They can be used to contaminate food or water sources, causing illness through ingestion.

WHAT THEY DO

Liquid nerve agents are rapidly absorbed into the skin, eyes, and lining of the mouth and if vaporized are absorbed primarily through the eyes and lungs.

Nerve agents disrupt the process of nerves communicating with other nerves or involuntary muscles (muscles that usually work without us thinking about them). Functions like salivating, sweating, control of pupils, urination, defecation, and breathing become overstimulated. In a concentrated exposure all of your muscles become unusable and flaccid (floppy) paralysis results. Death is usually due to respiratory failure from inability to use the muscles for breathing, obstruction of airflow from excessive secretions, or from heartbeat irregularities and dysfunction.

HOW DO YOU TELL WHAT IT IS?

Nerve agents are difficult to identify based on their characteristics alone, as they are usually colorless, odorless (or their smells vary), and tasteless. The most useful identification method would be noting the effects you and/or others around you are experiencing (see *SYMPTOMS* section below). Airborne chemicals could cause dead birds and insects to fall from the sky.

SARIN: Colorless, tasteless, and, as far as is known, odorless liquid. Sarin is the most volatile of all of the nerve agents, evaporating into the air at room temperature (72°F).
SOMAN: Colorless (or dark brown if aged) and tasteless liquid that has been variously described as smelling sweet, musty, fruity, spicy, nutty, or like camphor.
TABUN: Colorless and tasteless liquid, possibly having a faint fruity odor.
VX: Amber-colored, tasteless, and odorless oily liquid. It can be similar in appearance to motor oil.
GF: Very little information is available.

ASSESSMENT OF RISK

Risk of Use in an Attack

While the most deadly forms of nerve agents are available only to the armed forces, some commercial insecticides are similar to and approach the deadliness of weapons-grade chemicals. Many of these pesticides are readily available and are easier to obtain than their military counterparts.

The synthesizing of SARIN, TABUN, and SOMAN requires little expertise. SARIN and VX are both known to have been produced by terrorists in the past. SOMAN is more difficult to make than SARIN and TABUN. GF is made from chemicals that are fairly easy to obtain.

Though not impossible, using a gas as an effective weapon outdoors would require a very large amount to reach a number of people and would depend heavily upon weather conditions such as temperature, wind speed and direction, and humidity. In an enclosed space the effects could be much more deadly. It is considered unlikely that nerve agents would be used to contaminate food or water sources.

How Dangerous Are They?

Even one or two breaths from a very concentrated vapor exposure could produce loss of consciousness within seconds, followed by respiratory arrest, seizures, paralysis, and death within minutes.

SARIN: Sarin has an especially rapid onset of symptoms and is very deadly—it is 26 times more deadly than cyanide gas. A small drop of the liquid on the skin could be enough to cause death.
SOMAN: Soman is more deadly than both sarin and tabun.
TABUN: Tabun is one of the least lethal, gaseous nerve agents.
VX: VX is the most deadly of all of the nerve agents and also the least gaseous, meaning it is slower to evaporate. It is approximately 50 times more toxic than cyanide gas.
GF: It is reported that GF is less lethal than the others.

TIMELINE OF ILLNESS

For inhaled nerve agents, symptoms usually begin within seconds to minutes and death could occur in 1–10 minutes if enough chemical is inhaled. Maximal effects usually occur minutes after exposure stops. For liquid contact with the skin, reactions could be delayed, with symptoms occurring from 5 minutes to 18 hours following the time of exposure (the symptom-free period is usually 1–30 minutes); death could follow if exposure is concentrated enough.

Complete recovery could take several months. Severe exposure could cause permanent damage to the nervous system.

SYMPTOMS

INHALED MILD EXPOSURE: Sudden runny nose, watery eyes, shortness of breath, sneezing, sudden excess of saliva, headache, sweating, stomach cramps, nausea, twitching, tightness of the throat and chest. Most will have contraction (shrinking) of the pupils to the size of pinpoints (this could cause dimmed or blurred vision), though 13% may have dilated (enlarged) pupils.

INHALED CONCENTRATED EXPOSURE: May experience all of the mild symptoms with increased severity, in addition to drooling, spontaneous urination and/or release of stool, vomiting; blood-tinged saliva and nasal secretions; could cause sudden loss of consciousness, seizures, loss of all muscle control (a "floppy" paralysis, not a rigid or frozen muscle tone), wheezing, and respiratory failure from paralysis of the respiratory muscles.

SKIN EXPOSURE: Minimal exposure could cause sweating and twitching at the site of exposure; moderate exposure could cause upset stomach, vomiting, and diarrhea; significant exposure on the skin could cause loss of consciousness, seizures, paralysis, and respiratory failure from paralysis of respiratory muscles.

Nerve agents can also cause behavioral and psychological changes. These effects include irritability, nervousness, fatigue, insomnia, memory loss, impaired judgment, slurred speech, and depression.

EMERGENCY RESPONSE

- **Leave the exposure area at once** and seek fresh air.
- **Cover your nose and mouth** with a wet cloth.
- **Try not to breathe in** until you are out of the area of exposure; if you must breathe, take shallow breaths.
- **Try to remain calm.** Exposure may cause the production of large amounts of mucus and saliva and breathing may be difficult. Staying calm will help keep your airways open.
- **The antidotes atropine and pralidoxime should be administered as soon as possible** by trained professionals (see *TREATMENT* section below).
- **Start treatment and respiratory support quickly;** survival depends on it.
- **Nerve agents are heavier than air:** Do ***not*** go below ground level; do ***not*** lie on the floor or ground.
- **Remove all clothing** right away if possible and place in sealed, double plastic bags. Remove and wash jewelry as well.
- **Shower immediately** with copious amounts of soap and water, as nerve agents penetrate clothing.
- **Wash eyes within minutes of liquid nerve agent exposure** to limit injury. Flush with water for 5–10 minutes by tilting head to one side, pulling eyelids apart with fingers, and pouring water slowly into the eyes.
- **Wash clothing with bleach.**
- Note that while gas masks or air-purifying respirators are required for emergency responders working at the scene, the use of gas masks is not recommended to the untrained due to the danger from improper use.

TESTING AND DIAGNOSIS

Patients suspected of nerve-gas exposure (whether they show symptoms or not) should have a blood sample taken to check for the red-blood-cell enzyme activity of acetylcholinesterase. Since nerve gases disable this enzyme, it is usually more than 70% inactivated in exposed patients.

A chest x-ray is recommended for cases of severe exposure.

TREATMENT

Unless people are obviously contaminated and appear wet, it would be acceptable to give them mouth-to-mouth resuscitation, although this opinion remains controversial (see *SPECIAL PRECAUTIONS* below).

Airway must be opened and secured. Oxygen would likely need to be administered as soon as possible. A **ventilator** (breathing machine) may be necessary for severe breathing difficulties.

The antidote **atropine**, which primarily dries up excess secretions, should be given immediately. Repeating atropine administration may be necessary.

Patients should also be treated with the antidote **pralidoxime**, which works against further muscle paralysis. This must be administered within minutes to a few hours after exposure in order to be effective and should be given even if the patient is not exhibiting symptoms. Even though pralidoxime might not be effective for SOMAN, treatment should not be postponed until confirmation of the specific agent is made.

Even after appropriate antidote therapy, patients should be observed for paralysis and other neurologic symptoms. Agitation and confusion can result from large doses of atropine.

Valium may be necessary to treat convulsions.

ANTIDOTE

The antidotes **atropine** and **pralidoxime** are issued to people such as military personnel who are in danger of attacks and emergency medical workers who would respond to an attack. Atropine is readily available and frequently used in emergency and hospital settings. Pralidoxime is in very short supply.

CHILDREN

Children do not always respond to chemicals in the same way that adults do. Different protocols for managing their care may be needed. For example, dosages of atropine would probably differ from adult dosages and need to be adjusted.

PREGNANCY

Data is limited on the effects of nerve agents on developing embryos or fetuses. In terms of antidote usage, since their administration may well mean the difference between life and death, the benefits would outweigh any deleterious effects.

SPECIAL PRECAUTIONS

Exposure to a nerve gas could be fatal in a matter of minutes. Leaving shelter to rescue or assist victims during an ongoing release could be a deadly decision. Bear in mind that there is likely little help the untrained could offer that would be of any value to a victim of this chemical agent.

People who are contaminated with certain chemical agents may pose a danger to those who give them mouth-to-mouth resuscitation, **particularly when dealing with VX**. It is difficult to determine this risk in an emergency situation when the particular agent or concentration of the exposure is unknown. If there is a confirmed nerve agent attack other than VX, unless people are obviously contaminated and appear wet, it would be acceptable to assist them (although this advice remains controversial). As a precautionary measure, a pocket resuscitation mask could be purchased, which is a curved, plastic cup that rests over the victim's mouth and has a short tube attached to blow into for the rescuer.

While humidity generally lessens the effects of nerve agents, warm temperatures, regardless of humidity, will increase them.

ENVIRONMENTAL DECONTAMINATION AND CLEANUP

SARIN, SOBAN, TABUN: Could remain toxic for 10 minutes to 24 hours in the summer and 2 hours to 3 days in the wintertime.
SOMAN and GF: Moderate persistency.
VX: Slower to disperse, VX could remain toxic for 2–7 days in the summer and 2 days to weeks in the wintertime.

Water works well in the decontamination process, but in the case of a thickened nerve agent, soap and a household bleach solution should be used as well. The decontamination process should be performed by trained professionals equipped with protective clothing and respiratory protection.

HOW YOU CAN PREPARE

Keep health-facility and emergency phone numbers readily available (see *ADDITIONAL RESOURCES* below and the *Public Resources and Contact Information* section of the book).

Though protective, a charcoal-activated gas mask would likely be impractical in the event of a nerve-gas attack. It weighs about 4 pounds, and you would have to carry it everywhere to be ready for a surprise strike. If you choose to purchase one for your home, you must read the instructions carefully and practice with it, as improper use will not protect you and could actually suffocate you. WARNING: Our medical experts do not recommend the use of gas masks except by trained professionals. Data from Israel shows that the incorrect use of gas masks has caused many fatalities.

ADDITIONAL RESOURCES
Agency for Toxic Substances and Disease Registry (ATSDR)
   www.atsdr.cdc.gov
American College of Physicians-American Society of Internal Medicine
   www.acponline.org/bioterro/nerve_gas.htm
Centers for Disease Control (CDC)
   www.state.sd.us/doh/bioterrorism/chemical%20agents.pdf
Centers for Disease Control: Chemical/Biological/Radiological Hotline
   for obtaining information
   Hotline: 888-246-2675
Centers for Disease Control: Soman fact sheet
   www.bt.cdc.gov/agent/nerve/soman/ctc0004.asp
Centers for Disease Control: Tabun fact sheet
   www.bt.cdc.gov/agent/nerve/tabun/ctc0002.asp
Centers for Disease Control: VX fact sheet
   www.bt.cdc.gov/agent/nerve/vx/ctc0006.asp
Federation of American Scientists
   www.fas.org/nuke/intro/cw/agent.htm
National Response Center: Chemical/Biological/Radiological Hotline
   for reporting incidents
   Hotline: 800-424-8802
State public-health locator for officials, agencies, and public hotlines
   www.statepublichealth.org
The Survival Guide: What to Do in a Biological, Chemical, or Nuclear
   Emergency website: For updates, supplementary information, and
   helpful links
   www.911guide.com
U.S. Army Medical Research Institute of Chemical Defense (USAMRICD)
   ccc.apgea.army.mil
   Phone: 410-436-2230
U.S. Army Soldier and Biological Chemical Command
   www.sbccom.army.mil/services/edu/tabun.htm

PULMONARY IRRITANTS

CHEMICAL AGENTS	TYPE
Phosgene, Chlorine, Diphosgene, Chloropicrin, Ammonia	Pulmonary irritants (also known as "choking agents")

CHARACTERISTICS

PHOSGENE and CHLORINE are gases at room temperature; phosgene is colorless and smells like newly mown hay or green corn, and chlorine is greenish-yellow and has a pungent smell; DIPHOSGENE and CHLOROPICRIN are liquids and can be a range of colors, and diphosgene can smell like newly mown hay or green corn

HOW YOU GET EXPOSED

Primarily inhaled; also absorbed through the skin and mucous membranes (nose, throat, and especially the eyes)

TIME FROM EXPOSURE TO ILLNESS

Usually rapid, though effects of CHLORINE may be delayed

MAJOR SYMPTOMS

INHALED: Early symptoms may be irritated, burning eyes and throat, throat spasms, chest pain and tightness, and shortness of breath. Acute lung injury may follow (a life-threatening condition of fluid-filled lungs), indicated by severe shortness of breath and frothy saliva coming from the mouth and/or nose
ACQUIRED THROUGH THE SKIN: Skin or eye contact with these agents may result in severe chemical burns

EMERGENCY RESPONSE

- Leave the area of exposure at once
- Cover your nose and mouth with a cloth (wet if possible)
- Try not to breathe in until you have left the area; if you have to breathe, take shallow breaths
- Unless it inhibits your escape, close your eyes
- Pulmonary irritants are heavier than air: Do *not* go below ground level; do *not* lie on the floor or ground
- Try to remain calm—it will benefit breathing ability
- Gas masks are required for emergency responders working at the scene; however, the use of gas masks by the untrained is not recommended due to the danger of improper use

TREATMENT

Bed rest, warmth, oxygen supplementation, and possibly asthma medication for constricted airways

POSSIBILITY OF DEATH

Can be very high with concentrated or prolonged exposure

ANTIDOTE

None

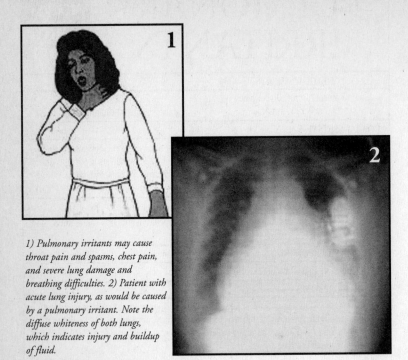

1) Pulmonary irritants may cause throat pain and spasms, chest pain, and severe lung damage and breathing difficulties. 2) Patient with acute lung injury, as would be caused by a pulmonary irritant. Note the diffuse whiteness of both lungs, which indicates injury and buildup of fluid.

WHAT THEY ARE

Pulmonary irritants are a group of chemicals that are also referred to as "respiratory" or "choking" agents because when inhaled their vapors primarily attack lung tissue, causing extensive damage as well as breathing difficulties. They are generally stored as liquids, but once a container is opened and they are exposed to the air, they rapidly become gases and expand to a wide area.

They have been used on the battlefield to incapacitate enemy troops. During World War I, because these gases are heavier than air, they would settle into foxholes and dugouts that troops would dive into, choking them in their own trenches. They were also used because they do not last long in the environment, so that troops arriving later would not be contaminated.

The lung-damaging agents that will be discussed in this chapter (followed by their military code names in parentheses) are PHOSGENE (CG), CHLORINE (CL), DIPHOSGENE (DP), CHLOROPICRIN (PS), and AMMONIA.

WHAT THEY DO

Pulmonary irritants are primarily absorbed by inhalation, with the severity of lung injury dependent upon the amount inhaled. For example, death can occur after inhaling only a few breaths of high concentrations of phosgene. For chlorine and chloropicrin, the windpipe may incur serious damage in addition to lung injury.

Once in the lungs the chemicals damage the tiny air sacs where we oxygenate blood, which leads to fluid buildup, which disrupts the vital exchange of oxygen. In severe cases the lungs eventually fill with these liquids and a person essentially drowns in his or her own body fluids.

Because most choking-agent chemicals are consumed by reactions in the lungs, they are not distributed throughout the body to any significant extent. Death occurs by respiratory failure.

HOW DO YOU TELL WHAT IT IS?

The presence of a choking agent would primarily be detected by the symptoms you and others around you experience. Rapid onset of burning in the throat, cough, chest discomfort, and breathing difficulty, particularly in addition to burning eyes, would suggest a possible choking-agent attack. The following includes general qualities for pure gases; note that these are not hard-and-fast indicators because the gases may well be mixed with other chemicals or substances that would change their characteristics:

PHOSGENE: Transported as a colorless liquid, phosgene gives off vapors that smell like green corn or newly mown hay. Upon explosion, a white cloud forms.
CHLORINE: Chlorine is a greenish-yellow gas with a pungent smell.
DIPHOSGENE: Diphosgene is a yellow to dark brown or black liquid and smells similar to phosgene (green corn or newly mown hay).
CHLOROPICRIN: Chloropicrin is a colorless to light green oily liquid at room temperature. Its specific smell is unknown.
AMMONIA (in the form of ANHYDROUS AMMONIA): A colorless liquid and vapor, this smells like ammonia used for household cleaning.

ASSESSMENT OF RISK

Risk of Use in an Attack

Although pulmonary irritants have not been used militarily since 1918, the risk of chlorine or phosgene as a terrorist weapon of choice remains because of their deadliness and their extensive use and availability in industry. The United States, for example, produces over a billion pounds of phosgene per year for industrial uses. Anhydrous ammonia (the type that would probably be used) is a common industrial refrigerant and is also used in the blueprinting process.

How Dangerous Is It?

Most of the pulmonary irritants can cause death within 10 minutes at very high concentrations.

If patients survive more than 48 hours after an acute exposure, they will usually recover fully. Chronic, low-concentration exposure could cause permanent lung damage.

TIMELINE OF ILLNESS

PHOSGENE: Onset of symptoms is rapid, beginning with irritation of the nose, eyes, and throat. Concentrated exposure could lead to death in 24–48 hours or less.
CHLORINE: Onset of symptoms following exposure could be rapid or take several hours. With moderate exposure, breathing could stop in 6–8 hours.
DIPHOSGENE: Onset of symptoms is rapid. With moderate exposure, breathing could stop in 6–8 hours.
CHLOROPICRIN: Onset of symptoms is very rapid. With moderate exposure, breathing could stop in 6–8 hours.
AMMONIA: Onset of symptoms is very rapid.

SYMPTOMS

In general, pulmonary irritants that have been inhaled cause severe damage to the lungs. Early symptoms may be irritated, burning eyes and throat; throat spasms; chest pain and tightness; and shortness of breath. Acute lung injury may follow, a life-threatening condition of fluid-filled lungs, indicated by severe shortness of breath and frothy sputum coming from the mouth and/or nose. Symptoms for phosgene are more detailed and apply to most of the other agents.

PHOSGENE: *Inhaled*—Early symptoms include irritation of the eyes, nose, and throat; cough; and chest pain. Spasms in the throat could cause death by asphyxiation (inability to get in oxygen). There may be a symptom-free period of up to 24 hours after low-dose exposure (this period could be shortened with physical exertion). Following this latent period, the most prominent symptom is shortness of breath, a result of an accumulation of fluid in the lungs, called acute lung injury; other signs of this condition are blood-tinged foam coming from the nose or mouth, nausea, vomiting, discomfort, restlessness, pale and clammy skin, low blood pressure, rapid heartbeat, and shock. Signs of acute lung injury within 4 hours of exposure indicate a low likelihood of survival for the patient. *Skin and Eyes*—Can burn eyes and skin; contact lesions may resemble frostbite or burns.

CHLORINE: *Inhaled*—Burning sensation, cough, headache, labored breathing, nausea, shortness of breath, sore throat. Acute lung injury may be delayed for a few symptom-free hours. *Skin and Eyes*—Can burn eyes and skin, causing pain, blurred vision, and severe deep burns.

DIPHOSGENE: *Inhaled*—Low-concentration exposure causes chest discomfort and/or shortness of breath. High concentrations quickly cause acute lung injury with cough, shortness of breath, and frothy sputum. Respiratory failure, low blood pressure, and death can follow. *Skin and Eyes*—Can burn and irritate skin. Tearing and irritation of the eyes; direct exposure can cause permanent damage to the corneas.

CHLOROPICRIN: *Inhaled*—Eyes tear, and nose and throat are irritated. Vapor exposure leads to coughing, difficulty breathing, sore throat, dizziness, bluish skin tone, vomiting, and possibly pulmonary edema. *Skin and Eyes*—Can cause chemical burns. Eyes may become red, teary, and painful. Prolonged exposure can cause blindness. With absorption through broken skin, symptoms may resemble those of inhalational exposure.

AMMONIA: **Inhaled**—Symptoms range from coughing to irritation to chemical pneumonia. *Skin and Eyes*—Can cause blisters and deep burns to the skin similar to frostbite. Most damaging to surface of the eye; initially causes severe pain and tearing, eventually causes corneal erosions, cloudy corneas, and cataract formation.

EMERGENCY RESPONSE

- **Leave the area of exposure immediately** and seek fresh air.

- **Try not to breathe in** before you are away from the vapors if you can; if you have to breathe, take shallow breaths.

- **Cover your nose and mouth with wet fabric.** Note that though gas masks and air-purifying respirators are required for emergency responders working at the scene, their use by the lay person is not recommended due to the danger of improper use.

- **Unless it inhibits your escape, close your eyes** until the vapors are gone.

- **Pulmonary irritants are heavier than air:** Do *not* go below ground level; do *not* lie on the floor or ground.

- **Flush eyes with water** for 15 minutes if exposed, removing contact lenses first and rolling eyes around beneath the stream of fluid. If you have persistent eye pain, call your doctor to see if you have corneal abrasions.
- **Try to remain calm**—it will benefit breathing ability.
- **If exposed, seek medical attention immediately**.

TESTING AND DIAGNOSIS

There are no available tests that readily diagnose human exposure to nerve agents. A chest x-ray after exposure would be abnormal, showing infiltration; a blood sample would show a high red-blood-cell count suggestive of hemoconcentration (low vascular fluid) and low oxygen. Lung-function tests would be abnormal.

TREATMENT

Asthma medication can be given to relieve spasms of the airways. Bronchodilators and steroids may also be used for bronchospasm.

Supplemental oxygen or a **ventilator** (breathing machine) may be required, which can be especially beneficial early on. Airway secretions must be cleared and managed.

Bed rest should be enforced, as increased activity will make respiratory symptoms more severe, which could lead to respiratory failure and death.

Tightness of the chest and coughing should also be treated with **comfortable warmth** (e.g., a blanket).

Intravenous fluids and **vasopressor medications** should be administered to increase low blood pressure if necessary.

ANTIDOTE

None exists.

CHILDREN

The above medications are safe for children, but dosages should be adjusted.

PREGNANCY

The above medications are safe for pregnant women.

SPECIAL PRECAUTIONS

Exposure to a pulmonary irritant could be fatal. Leaving shelter to rescue or assist victims during an ongoing release could be a deadly decision. Bear in mind that there is likely little help the untrained could offer that would be of any value to a victim of this chemical agent.

Although bleach is recommended to decontaminate for other agents, mixing bleach and AMMONIA could be dangerous.

ENVIRONMENTAL DECONTAMINATION AND CLEANUP

Because of their tendency to evaporate, pulmonary irritants would not remain in the liquid form for long (see below), hence environmental decontamination would not be required unless they were used in very cold climates or combined with a thickening agent to make the irritant more persistent. For the latter scenarios, water would probably be used to hose off the area. For CHLORINE, which could remain for a day or two, the area might be barricaded until it was safe or water would be used to hose off the area.

Persistence in the Environment

PHOSGENE: 40–60°F is 1 hour, 70–90°F is 30 minutes
CHLORINE: 40–60°F is 2–3 days, 70–90°F is 18–36 hours
DIPHOSGENE: 40–60°F is 1–4 hours, 70–90°F is 30 minutes to 3 hours

HOW YOU CAN PREPARE

Keep health-facility and emergency phone numbers readily available (see *ADDITIONAL RESOURCES* below and the *Public Resources and Contact Information* section of the book).

While a gas mask would protect the eyes and airways from pulmonary-irritant fumes, one would have to have immediate access to one. It weighs about 4 pounds, and you would have to carry it everywhere to be ready for a surprise strike. If you choose to purchase one for your home, you must read the instructions carefully and practice using it, as improper use will not protect you and could actually suffocate you. WARNING: Our medical experts do not recommend the use of gas masks except by trained professionals. Data from Israel shows that the incorrect use of gas masks has caused many fatalities.

Protective clothing is not readily needed because the predominant entry for pulmonary irritants is inhalation.

ADDITIONAL RESOURCES

Centers for Disease Control (CDC)
www.state.sd.us/doh/bioterrorism/chemical%20agents.pdf
Centers for Disease Control: Chemical/Biological/Radiological Hotline
for obtaining information
Hotline: 888-246-2675
Federation of American Scientists
www.fas.org/nuke/intro/cw/agent.htm
National Response Center: Chemical/Biological/Radiological Hotline
for reporting incidents
Hotline: 800-424-8802
State public-health locator for officials, agencies, and public hotlines
www.statepublichealth.org
The Survival Guide: What to Do in a Biological, Chemical, or Nuclear
Emergency website: For updates, supplementary information, and
helpful links
www.911guide.com
U.S. Army Medical Research Institute of Chemical Defense (USAMRICD)
ccc.apgea.army.mil
Phone: 410-436-2230

UNIDENTIFIED CHEMICAL AGENT

CHEMICAL AGENT	TYPE
Unidentified	Chemical gas, liquid, or powder

POSSIBLE EARLY SYMPTOMS

May include burning eyes, nose, or throat; burning skin; excessive salivation; runny eyes; profuse mucus production in nasal passages and airways, possibly blood-tinged; extremely dry mouth; fluid-filled blisters; welts (like bee stings); rashes; pinpoint or dilated pupils; difficulty breathing; chest pain; choking; nausea; vomiting; involuntary release of urine or stool; changes in skin color; headache; dimmed or blurred vision; dizziness; disorientation; unusual behavior; lack of coordination; trembling; convulsions; paralysis; and/or loss of consciousness

EMERGENCY RESPONSE

- Leave the area of exposure at once; seconds may count
- Don't touch suspicious substances
- Go against the wind and uphill; do not go below ground unless instructed otherwise
- Cover your nose and mouth with fabric (wet if possible)
- Breathe as little as possible until out of the exposure area; take shallow breaths if necessary
- Close your eyes if it does not inhibit escape
- Remove clothing and rinse skin with lots of water (shower if possible), even if symptom-free
- Flush eyes with water for 10–15 minutes
- Seek medical attention immediately if you may have been exposed to a chemical agent
- Gas masks or air-purifying respirators may be required for emergency responders working at the scene of a chemical attack; the use of gas masks by the untrained is not recommended due to the danger of improper use
- Be prepared to evacuate, or alternatively, to shelter-in-place

TREATMENT

The primary treatment for most chemical agents is antidotes and should begin as soon as possible; if available, they are administered by emergency professionals on the scene

ANTIDOTE

Because of the rapid action of many chemical agents, antidote treatment may be initiated based on symptoms before the agent's identity is confirmed

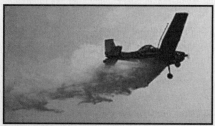

Chemical agents, as well as biological or even radiological agents, could be disseminated via a low-flying crop-duster plane

OVERVIEW

Of all of the chemical-weapons chapters in this book, this may be one of the most important to read, as the most likely scenario to occur would be an emergency situation in which people are falling ill from an unknown agent. In other words, you would need to act before all of the evidence was in.

Chemical agents may be solids, liquids, or gases; some have colors and odors, while others are completely undetectable and cannot be seen or smelled. They could be dispersed in many ways, most likely via airborne sprays or weapons or by coating surfaces with oily liquids. They could be sprayed as solids or liquids, used to contaminate a ventilation system, or placed as a liquid to vaporize among crowds. For example, in the Tokyo subways in 1995, a Japanese cult used packages containing the nerve agent sarin, which vaporized into airborne poison; 12 people died and more than 5,000 were injured. In the late 1980s Iraq used bombs that appear to have leaked nerve- and blister-agent gases upwind of a Kurdish village, killing hundreds.

It is not necessary for terrorists to build complicated chemical release devices, however—other alternatives are sabotaging or bombing a chemical plant and letting the toxic cloud drift into a populated area. They could also attack freight trains or highway trucks carrying hazardous materials.

NATIONAL, STATE, AND LOCAL RESPONSES TO AN ATTACK

As in the event of any emergency, state or local officials will be responsible for the initial response with support from federal agencies such as the Environmental Protection Agency (EPA), Federal Emergency Management Authority (FEMA), and Department of Transportation (DOT). The Centers for Disease Control (CDC) responds to all public-health emergencies, including chemical emergencies, whether caused by an act of terrorism or an accidental release.

It is the state and local public-health professionals who work alongside the local police, firefighters, and emergency medical personnel in affected areas. An incident commander will be assigned and the appropriate emergency personnel will be dispatched. Generally a local hazardous material (or "Haz-Mat") team, specially trained in dealing with chemical emergencies, will respond. During an event, it is very important that you follow the instructions of these highly trained professionals.

The first objective of emergency responders on the scene will be to identify the chemical. This may be an easy task since all chemical containers are required to identify their substance and all vehicles transporting chemicals are required to have placards that identify the substance and its properties.

In the event of a terrorist act, however, identifying the substance may prove to be a formidable challenge. Depending on the type and the amount of chemical released, the team will try to minimize the dispersal of the chemical in one or more ways: they may use water, sand, dirt, foam, or other materials to dilute the chemical and keep it from spreading outside the immediate zone of release. All emergency personnel will be wearing protective clothing and using self-contained breathing apparatuses (SCBAs) to keep them as safe as possible during their operations.

TIMELINE OF ILLNESS

Chemical agents can cause illness anywhere from seconds to days after exposure. Most cause symptoms very rapidly, within no more than a couple of hours.

INDICATORS OF A POSSIBLE CHEMICAL INCIDENT

Indicators of a chemical incident include **mass casualties** (numerous individuals exhibiting unexplained serious health problems, including incapacitation, convulsions, and death), **numerous individuals experiencing similar, unexplained symptoms** (see table above, *Possible Early Symptoms*), **casualties distributed in a pattern** that may be associated with possible agent dissemination methods, **illness associated within a confined geographic area** (such as most victims are in a certain building or most are outdoors within a certain area); **dead animals, birds, fish, or insects** (birds and insects may fall from the sky); **vegetation dies out of season**, unexplained by weather conditions; **unusual liquid droplets** (numerous hard surfaces exhibit oily droplets or film and no recent rain; water surfaces have an oily film); **unexplained odors** (especially fruity, flowery, sharp/pungent, garlic, horseradish, bitter almonds, peach kernels, or newly mown hay smells; it is important to note that the particular odor is completely out of character with surroundings); **low-lying clouds or foglike atmosphere** unexplained by weather, smog, or the surroundings; **unusual metal debris** (unexplained bomb/munitions material, especially if it is wet and there has been no recent rain). (From *"Chemical/Biological/Radiological Incident Handbook,"* by the Chemical, Biological and Radiological (CBRN) Subcommittee, 1998.)

See also Chapter 16, *Unidentified Biological Agent*, **Table 2**, Comparison of Biological and Chemical Weapons.

TESTING AND DIAGNOSIS

When emergency personnel, such as the hazardous materials ("Haz-Mat") team, arrive, they will have test kits that can identify a variety of chemicals on the spot. However, if they are not able to confirm the exact substance right away, action must be taken nonetheless because many chemical agents cause effects so rapidly. Diagnoses may be made based upon symptom patterns of victims.

TREATMENT

Treatments for chemical agents are usually antidotes, antitoxins, and other neutralizing agents and should begin immediately. Most are by prescription only and need to be administered by trained professionals. Emergency personnel on the scene will tell you what to do and advise you on decontamination procedures.

ANTIDOTE

Antidotes are available for some nerve agents, blister agents, and chemical asphyxiants ("blood agents"), as well as Agent 15. The determination to use these will be made by onsite emergency personnel.

CHILDREN

- Because many of the chemicals that might be used in a terrorist attack are heavier than air, children might be disproportionately affected merely because they are closer to the ground.
- For their body weight, children have a greater skin surface area than adults, which could expose them more to blister agents, such as mustard gas.
- Children breathe faster than adults, which could potentially put them at more risk for inhalational chemical agents.
- Dosages of antidotes must be adjusted.

PREGNANCY

- There are no special precautions for pregnant women for most chemical agents or their treatments.
- Data on the effects of antidote usage on a developing fetus is limited, but if its administration meant the difference between life and death, the benefits would outweigh possible deleterious effects.
- If it is later determined that a blister agent attack has occurred, post-exposure counseling to the pregnant woman is very important, as this agent may cause severe developmental abnormalities to a developing fetus.

SPECIAL PRECAUTIONS

You may be asked to **shelter-in-place** for a period of time:

- The safest place in your home would be an above-ground inner room without windows.
- Turn off any ventilation systems and close doors, windows, and fireplace dampers.

- If you are instructed to seal your windows, doors, and vents (including air-conditioning units, bathroom and kitchen exhaust fans, and stove and dryer vents) with duct tape and plastic sheeting (or wax paper or aluminum foil), be sure to maintain enough ventilation to prevent suffocation.
- Keep water, food with a long shelf life, bedding, medicines, and anything else you may need for at least a 3-day stay in the shelter room (see Chapter 33, *Preparedness and Response Supplies,* for more suggestions on what to store).
- Listen to your television or radio until you are told it is safe to come out or that you must evacuate.

If you are told to **evacuate** immediately:

- Take your evacuation kit with you (see Chapter 33).
- Do not assume emergency shelters will have everything you need— in most cases they provide only emergency items such as meals, cots, and blankets.
- Follow exact evacuation instructions from authorities: taking alternate routes may put you in danger.
- Close your car windows and air vents and turn off the heater or air-conditioner.

As it can only take seconds to become affected by some chemical agents, leaving shelter during an ongoing release to rescue or assist victims could be a deadly decision. Bear in mind that there is likely little or no help the untrained could offer that would be of any value to a victim of a chemical agent. Further, touching the body of a contaminated person could bring the poison into your own body.

People who are contaminated with certain chemical agents may pose a danger to those who give them mouth-to-mouth resuscitation. It is difficult to determine this risk in an emergency situation when the particular agent or concentration of the exposure is unknown. As a precautionary measure, a pocket resuscitation mask could be purchased; this is a curved plastic cup that rests over the victim's mouth and has a short tube attached for the rescuer to blow into.

ENVIRONMENTAL DECONTAMINATION AND CLEANUP

- Be wary of chemical residue in the area of the attack. Follow instructions from emergency officials concerning cleanup methods. Local officials will best know proper procedures for your particular situation.
- Follow local instructions concerning the safety of food and water. Contaminated food or water can cause illness.

HOW YOU CAN PREPARE

Keep health-facility and emergency phone numbers readily available (see *ADDITIONAL RESOURCES* below and the *Public Resources and Contact Information* section of the book).

Over-the-counter items that may be useful in a chemical attack:
   Activated charcoal
   Antihistamines
   Betadine (povodine iodine)
   Eye wash (0.9% saline solution)
   Household liquid chlorine bleach (sodium hypochlorite,
        5%) without other ingredients; to formulate a 0.5%
        bleach solution, mix 1 part bleach to 9 parts water
   Pocket resuscitation mask

Note that a charcoal-activated gas mask, while protective for most chemical agents, would likely be impractical in the event of an attack. It weighs about 4 pounds, and you would have to carry it everywhere to be ready for a surprise strike. If you choose to purchase one for your home, you must read the instructions carefully and practice with it, as improper use will not protect you and could actually suffocate you. WARNING: Our medical experts do not recommend the use of gas masks except by trained professionals. Data from Israel shows that the incorrect use of gas masks has caused many fatalities.

ADDITIONAL RESOURCES

American Red Cross
    www.redcross.org/services/disaster/keepsafe/chemical.html#after
Centers for Disease Control (CDC)
    www.state.sd.us/doh/bioterrorism/chemical%20agents.pdf
Centers for Disease Control: Chemical/Biological/Radiological Hotline
    for obtaining information: 888-246-2675
Federal Emergency Management Agency (FEMA)
    www.fema.gov Phone: 202-646-4600
Metropolitan Medical Response System (MMRS)
    www.mmrs.hhs.gov
National Response Center: Chemical/Biological/Radiological Hotline
    for reporting incidents: 800-424-8802
State public-health locator for officials, agencies, and public hotlines
    www.statepublichealth.org
U.S. Army Medical Research Institute of Chemical Defense (USAMRICD)
    ccc.apgea.army.mil Phone: 410-436-2230

EARLY INDICATORS OF CHEMICAL AGENT EXPOSURE

The presence of a chemical agent would primarily be detected by the symptoms you and others around you were experiencing.

CHEMICAL	Most Likely Form	Common Odor	Common Color	Onset of Symptoms	Early Symptoms	Weight Compared to Air*
NERVE AGENTS						
Sarin	Liquid / vapor	Odorless	Colorless	Rapid	From vapor release, runny nose, watery eyes, shortness of breath, sweating, sneezing, dimmed or blurred vision, red eyes, drooling, pinpoint pupils (though sometimes dilated)	Heavier
Soman	Liquid / vapor	Sweet, musty, fruity spicy, nutty, or like camphor	Colorless or dark brown	Seconds to minutes if inhaled, 5 min–18 hrs from skin contact with liquid	Same as above	Heavier
Tabun	Liquid / vapor	Faintly fruity	Colorless	Seconds to minutes if inhaled, 5 min–18 hrs from skin contact with liquid	Same as above	Heavier
VX	Oily liquid	Odorless	Amber (colorless if pure)	Seconds to minutes if inhaled, 5 min–18 hrs from skin contact with liquid	Same as above	Heavier
BLISTER AGENTS						
Mustard Gas	Gas	Garlic, mustard, or onion; or could be nearly odorless	Range—could be colorless, shades of yellow, brown or black	Possibly delayed for hours to days	Burning of the skin, large blisters form on the skin, eye and airway irritation, sore throat, cough, chest pain, profuse mucus in nasal passages and airways, nausea and vomiting can also occur	Heavier
Lewisite	Oily liquid	Odorless or like geraniums	Colorless or amber to dark brown	Immediate	Same as above	Heavier
Phosgene Oxime	Solid or liquid	Pepper with unpleasant, pungent odor	Colorless	Immediate	Hives or welts, but no blisters form on skin	Heavier

EARLY INDICATORS OF CHEMICAL AGENT EXPOSURE *continued*

The presence of a chemical agent would primarily be detected by the symptoms you and others around you were experiencing.

CHEMICAL	Most Likely Form	Common Odor	Common Color	Onset of Symptoms	Early Symptoms	Weight Compared to Air*
PULMONARY IRRITANTS ("CHOKING AGENTS")						
Phosgene	Liquid / vapor	Green corn or newly mown hay	Colorless	Rapid; respiratory symptoms could be delayed for 20 minutes—24 hours after low dose	From inhalation, irritated burning eyes and throat, throat spasms, chest pain, shortness of breath. Skin/eye contact may cause severe chemical burns.	Heavier
Chlorine	Gas	Pungent smell	Greenish-yellow	Could be rapid or delayed up to several hours	From inhalation, irritated burning eyes and throat, cough, headache, shortness of breath, nausea. Skin/eye contact may cause severe chemical burns.	Heavier
Diphosgene	Liquid	Green corn or newly mown hay	Range from yellow to dark brown or black	Rapid	From inhalation, chest discomfort, shortness of breath. Skin contact may cause irritation, eye contact can result in permanent damage.	Heavier
Chloropicrin	Oily liquid	Intense and penetrating	Colorless to light green	Very rapid	From inhalation, irritated burning eyes, nose and coughing, difficulty breathing, dizziness, vomiting. Skin/eye contact may cause severe chemical burns.	Heavier
Ammonia	Liquid / vapor	Sharp and caustic	Colorless	Very rapid	Burns eyes, blisters skin, burns lungs if inhaled	Heavier
CHEMICAL ASPHYXIANTS ("BLOOD AGENTS")						
Hydrogen Cyanide	Gas or liquid	Bitter almonds	Colorless	Very rapid	Mild irritation to eyes, nose, and airways; shortness of breath, agitation, weakness, nausea, vomiting, muscular trembling; convulsions; respiratory arrest	Lighter
Cyanogen Chloride	Gas	Bitter almonds	Colorless	Rapid	Same as above, with greater burning sensation to eyes, throat, and lungs	Heavier
Arsine	Gas	Garlic	Colorless	30—60 minutes, or delayed for several hours	Red eyes, garlic breath odor, headache, thirst, shivering, weakness, abdominal pain	Lighter

* If a chemical is heavier than air, it will sink when delivered as a vapor. In these cases, one should *not* go below ground level or lie on the floor or ground. When a chemical is lighter than air, it would be expected to rise after a vapor release.

RADIATION PRIMER

This chapter is intended to offer a more in-depth explanation of (1) what radiation is and why it is harmful, (2) the radioactive risks of dirty bombs, (3) what nuclear weapons are, how they work, and what their capabilities are, and (4) how nuclear reactors work and the radioactive dangers they bear.

RADIATION

Most atoms are stable and are therefore nonradioactive. Those that have unstable nuclei—such as uranium and radium—will disintegrate and give off energy in the form of elementary particles and rays. Radiation is the process of emitting energy. Small quantities of radiation occur naturally in the air we breathe, the water we drink, and the food we eat. We are also exposed to radiation from diagnostic medical procedures such as x-rays, and in the form of cosmic rays from the sun and other stars in the galaxy. Ionizing radiation is a type of radiation that is harmful to human tissues. Dirty bombs, nuclear bombs, and nuclear-reactor leaks or explosions would give off varying levels and types of ionizing radiation, and the effects on a living organism would vary based on these differences.

There are two different types of radiation: particulate (such as α and β particles) and electromagnetic (which occurs in waves). For electromagnetic radiation there is a relationship between energy and wavelength, which is that as the wavelength decreases, energy increases. Going from the longest wavelength and lowest energy (and least harmful) to the shortest and highest, we have radio waves, microwaves, infrared light, visible light, ultraviolet (UV) rays, x-rays and gamma (γ) rays. The latter two can penetrate deep into the body.

The Four Most Common Forms of Ionizing Radiation

Alpha (α) particles: The weakest particles, they can penetrate only air and can be stopped by a sheet of paper. Because they are large, they cannot travel far and cannot penetrate past the top, dead layers of our skin or clothing. Thus they pose no hazard outside of our bodies, but if inhaled or ingested they could cause severe internal injury. They would be a fallout hazard in the event of a nuclear bomb.

Beta (β) particles: Beta particles are very light and hence can travel farther than alpha particles. They can penetrate skin in large enough quantities to cause a thermal burn (also called a "beta burn") and can penetrate up to a millimeter of lead. They are primarily found in fallout radiation in the event of a nuclear bomb.

Gamma (γ) rays: Gamma rays are bursts of photons (particles of electro-magnetic energy) that can penetrate up to 3 inches of lead. They are emitted in a nuclear detonation and fallout. They are similar to x-rays, which are also electromagnetic but are generated in electronic devices rather than in nuclear processes. Because of their high energy and penetrative capabilities, gamma rays are very harmful to humans.

Neutrons (η): Neutrons have significant mass and energy, and because they interact with nuclei of other atoms, they cause severe disruption of other atomic structures. In fact, neutrons are extremely penetrative and can cause 20 times more damage to tissue than gamma rays for the same deposited total dose of energy. Neutrons are only emitted during a nuclear detonation or part of a nuclear reactor leak. They are not a fallout hazard.

Radiological Effects of Ionizing Radiation on the Human Body

Ionizing radiation injures cells by interacting with critical molecules within them. At high doses (above 2 sieverts) this can result in cell death, organ damage, and even death to the individual. (Note: Most people receive about 3.33 millisieverts [1 millisievert = 1/1000 of a sievert] per year from natural exposure.) This is called "direct damage." Cells can also be injured indirectly by radiation interaction with water molecules in the body, leading to the formation of toxic molecules that in turn cause cellular damage.

When the body is exposed to a high level of radiation, a serious illness called **acute radiation sickness (ARS)** can occur. Symptoms may begin within minutes to hours. Many survivors of the Hiroshima and Nagasaki atomic bombs of the 1940s and the emergency responders of the Chernobyl nuclear power-plant accident in 1986 became ill with ARS.

Cells that are most sensitive to radiation effects are the rapidly dividing cells of the bone marrow and gastrointestinal tracts. Recovery from cellular injury after radiation exposure is possible but there remains a higher than normal probability of developing later cancers or mutations.

If radiation damage occurs in the genes (which are made up of DNA), cancer may occur later in life. Most of the time when DNA becomes damaged the body is able to repair it, but if the damaged DNA is not repaired, cells can turn cancerous. Cancer results from cells losing their ability to regulate their rate of division and thus they reproduce uncontrollably. If the genetic damage occurs in sperm or eggs, then hereditary mutations may be passed on to offspring.

Radiation is not as great a carcinogen as many people fear, however. People who survived the effects of radiation of a nuclear blast would probably have an increased cancer risk of only 15% (35% versus 20% baseline for unexposed people), as demonstrated by survivors of the Hiroshima and Nagasaki bombs. There is some evidence that external exposure—such as that received by survivors of Hiroshima and Nagasaki—is not as dangerous as internal—such as that experienced by cleanup workers at Chernobyl who either died or have now passed on increased mutations to their offspring.

DIRTY BOMBS

A "dirty bomb" is a device that uses conventional explosives like dynamite to scatter radioactive material. Sources of material could be radioactive waste or used fuel rods from a nuclear power plant, though these are heavily guarded by nuclear facilities. A dirty bomb would more than likely incorporate relatively available radioactive material, such as cesium-137 or cobalt-60, which could be stolen from places like hospitals. It would not result in the type of radioactive plume associated with a nuclear bomb or Chernobyl-type accident. It is unlikely that the radioactive material in a dirty bomb would kill anyone.

NUCLEAR BOMBS

"Nuclear bomb" and "nuclear weapon" are general terms that can refer to an ATOMIC, HYDROGEN, or NEUTRON BOMB. Atomic bombs were developed first. These were the type of bombs dropped over the Japanese cities of Hiroshima and Nagasaki to end World War II. Hydrogen bombs, developed about 10 years later, are about 500 times or more powerful than atomic bombs; they have thus far never been used in warfare, only in testing. Neutron bombs, developed most recently, are nuclear weapons that minimize damage to buildings and equipment but maximize damage to people. All of the above use the process of fission, fusion, or a combination of both to achieve their effects.

Fission Weapons

Fission is basically a nuclear reaction in which nuclei of atoms are bombarded by neutrons and split in two, releasing large amounts of energy and creating a chain reaction of nuclei splitting. **Uranium** is often the fuel used since it can be readily fabricated into a fissionable weapon. **Plutonium** is also used. Called ATOMIC BOMBS, fission weapons have an explosive yield measured in kilotons (1 kiloton = 1,000 tons of TNT). They produce radioactive fallout if the detonation occurs close enough to land or water. The power of these bombs is enormous. For example, the atomic bomb dropped on Hiroshima used 855 grams of highly enriched uranium, had a yield of 12.5 kilotons, killed 70,000 people instantaneously, and after 5 years caused a total death toll of around 200,000; the bomb used at Nagasaki contained 13 pounds of plutonium, had a yield of 21 kilotons, and killed 40,000 people and after 5 years around 150,000 total.

Fusion Weapons

Fusion is essentially the process in which two nuclei combine, or "fuse" together, at extremely high temperature to form a heavier nucleus, releasing large amounts of energy. The fusion of hydrogen atoms—two isotopes of hydrogen most readily fused together are hydrogen-2 (**deuterium**) and hydrogen-3 (**tritium**)—produces helium.

Fusion is the process that occurs in HYDROGEN (also known as THERMONUCLEAR) BOMBS. This is also the process that powers the sun. The explosive yield of hydrogen bombs is measured in megatons (1 megaton = 1,000,000 tons of TNT). For example, the first hydrogen bomb tested in the United States, in 1952, was 10 megatons (over 500 times more powerful than the bomb used on Hiroshima). Hydrogen bombs can be hundreds or thousands of times more powerful than atomic bombs and can be made small enough to fit in warheads of intercontinental ballistic missiles. One worst-case scenario estimated that a 1-megaton explosion in Detroit could kill 250,000 people, injure half a million more, and flatten all buildings within a 1.7-mile radius.

Fission/Fusion Combination Weapons

All nuclear weapons that are not pure fission weapons use fusion reactions to enhance their destructive effects. Weapons that use fusion require a fission bomb to provide the energy and extremely high heat (reaching the temperature of the interior of stars) to initiate the fusion reactions. The largest nuclear explosion ever set off was 50 megatons and called the Tsar Bomba (King of Bombs), a Soviet fission-fusion-fission design. It was tested in 1961 over an island in the Arctic Sea.

The NEUTRON BOMB, also called an "enhanced radiation warhead," is a specialized type of small thermonuclear weapon that uses a fission explosion to begin a fusion reaction. It produces minimal blast and heat (confined to a few hundred yards) but releases large amounts of lethal radiation. Within a somewhat larger area it throws off a massive wave of neutron and gamma radiation that can penetrate armor or several feet of earth. This radiation is extremely destructive to living tissue.

NUCLEAR POWER PLANTS (NUCLEAR REACTORS)

How They Work

If the chain reaction of **fission** is controlled and gradual, it can be harnessed and used to make electricity in a nuclear power plant. The reaction itself takes place in a **nuclear fuel rod**, a long metal rod that contains ceramic pellets of enriched uranium or plutonium. These fuel rods rest in a bundle in the nuclear reactor and are submerged in water inside a pressure vessel. The nuclear reaction acts as an extremely high-energy source of heat. The heat then turns the water into steam, which drives a steam turbine, which in turn spins a generator to produce power.

Safety Measures

The reactor's pressure vessel typically has a concrete liner that acts as a radiation shield. That liner is housed within a much larger steel containment vessel, which is intended to prevent leakage of any radioactive gases or fluids from the plant. The containment vessel is also usually protected by a second containment structure—an outer concrete building that is 2–5 feet thick, reinforced with steel, and strong enough to survive such things as hurricanes and small plane crashes. Secondary containment structures are necessary to prevent the escape of radiation/radioactive steam in the event of an accident.

Nuclear power plants have many safety systems to protect workers, the public, and the environment. These include shutting the reactor down quickly and stopping the fission process, systems to cool the reactor down and carry heat away from it, and barriers to contain the radioactivity and prevent it from escaping into the environment.

A Nuclear Power-Plant Meltdown, Leak, or Explosion

With any nuclear reactor, there is the possibility of a malfunction that could cause the nuclear chain reaction to run out of control, resulting in extremely high temperatures and a **meltdown** of the fuel rods. Meltdowns that breach a reactor containment vessel could potentially release huge amounts of radiation into the surrounding environment. Following a major accident, along with the initial radiation exposure, the land and water covering a large area around an accident site could become contaminated and unfit for human habitation for hundreds of years.

A nuclear plant cannot blow up like a nuclear bomb because a power plant does not keep its uranium or plutonium compact enough to set off the intense and rapid chain reaction needed for a bomb explosion. A nuclear-reactor leak or explosion, however, would pose a significant radioactive risk to the immediately surrounding and even more distant inhabitants. People caught under the initial and nearby passing radioactive fallout cloud from a reactor accident could be exposed to large doses of harmful gamma rays and potentially lethal radiation sickness. Inhalation and ingestion of other radioactive gases and particles could cause cancers and diseases in the lungs, digestive system, blood, and reproductive organs.

Nuclear reactors' highly radioactive waste (the **used fuel rods** known as "spent fuel") is kept cool in pools of water inside the plant. It could ignite if exposed to air and possibly cause a catastrophic fire worse than a reactor meltdown.

After the Chernobyl reactor exploded in the former USSR (now Ukraine) in 1986, it burned for days before it was extinguished. The absence of a secondary containment structure allowed radioactive material to escape. Thus, particles of highly radioactive irradiated fuel were lofted into a plume, which then created fallout locally and over much of Europe. The radioactivity eventually circled the Northern Hemisphere several times. Many of the workers and cleanup workers from Chernobyl have died, and an increased rate of illness and cancer in the area is attributed to the accident, especially among children exposed.

Fallout

Radioactive iodine-131 is generated in nuclear power plants and is a major health concern in an airborne release from a damaged reactor because of its mobility, radioactivity, persistence in the environment, and rapid uptake into the human body. In this case, potassium iodide is the appropriate emergency treatment for those in the vicinity (at least within a 10-mile radius). A release would also contain radioactive fallout of other radioactive substances such as cesium-137 and strontium-90, each with an approximate half-life of 30 years (the time required for half of the material to transform or decay). These radioactive elements can be incorporated into body tissues, particularly bone, and cause harmful effects years after their uptake.

DIRTY BOMBS

RADIOACTIVE EVENT

Dirty Bomb

DESCRIPTION

Radioactive substance with conventional explosive

TIME FROM EXPOSURE TO ILLNESS

Minutes to years, though most injuries would be due to the explosion itself

MAJOR SYMPTOMS

Though acute radiation poisoning after a dirty bomb detonation is extremely unlikely, symptoms include upset stomach, vomiting, diarrhea, skin burns, peeling skin, weakness, fatigue, dehydration, inflammation, hair loss, open sores on the skin and in the mouth or along intestinal tract, vomiting blood, bloody stool, and bleeding from the nose, mouth, and gums

EMERGENCY RESPONSE

- Leave the area of the blast site as quickly as possible, going against the wind if possible
- Cover your mouth and nose with fabric (wet if possible) if in the immediate area
- Seek shelter; go to a basement without windows if possible or else an inner room
- Unless you have been directed to a decontamination site by public-health officials, remove clothing and shower
- Avoid mass transit; leave the immediate area on foot (if you take a private vehicle, you might contaminate it)
- Listen to the radio or television for instructions from emergency officials
- Be prepared to evacuate

TREATMENT

Potassium iodide if radioactive iodine is confirmed (unlikely)

POSSIBILITY OF DEATH

High from explosion, low from radioactivity

WHAT IT IS

A dirty bomb—also known as a radiological dispersal device (RDD)—combines conventional explosives, like dynamite, with radioactive materials, such as from used nuclear reactor fuel rods or hospital stores of radionuclides and isotopes. It is

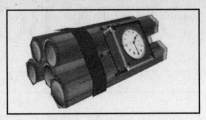

Dirty bombs pair conventional explosives, like dynamite, with radioactive materials.

designed to spread radioactive material around an area the size of a few city blocks. The radioactive substance would probably be in the form of pellets or powder. It is not a nuclear bomb and does not involve a nuclear explosion.

Experts believe a dirty bomb could range in size from a small "suitcase" device to a truck bomb, and could be larger.

WHAT IT DOES

Effects from a Bomb Blast

Explosives produce four main effects:

Blast pressure. The explosion creates a pressure wave that extends in all directions away from the blast, followed by a vacuum created by this wave. People near the blast can be thrown by the wave and then pulled back toward the blast by the vacuum, suffering injuries similar to those sustained in a car accident. A large enough pressure wave would immediately disintegrate a human body.

Fragmentation. Damage due to flying objects, including fragments from the bomb itself.

Thermal effects. Damage due to heat and fire.

Seismic shock. Ground movement in the event of large detonations (such as the Oklahoma City bombing).

Radiological Effects

Radiation kills or damages rapidly dividing cells such as blood-forming cells found in the bone marrow and cells that line the intestinal tract. Severe exposure results in "radiation poisoning," causing untreated victims to dehydrate and bleed to death, although there is very little chance of this happening after a dirty-bomb explosion. The disruption of normal cell functioning that radiation causes can sometimes lead to cancer many years later.

CAN YOU TELL IF A BOMB IS RADIOACTIVE?

Radiological materials are colorless, odorless, and tasteless and cannot be detected by humans without specialized equipment. Thus, one should assume there is radioactivity present if near a blast and take the necessary precautions (see *EMERGENCY RESPONSE* below).

ASSESSMENT OF RISK

Risk of Use in an Attack

Despite the fact that use of chemical and biological weapons is on the rise, bombings are still used in approximately 70% of all acts of terrorism. The main reasons for this are:

1) They are cheap to make.
2) The components to make them, such as bags of fertilizer, are widely available.
3) The instant a bomb detonates it creates public fear and draws media attention, which are a terrorist's goals in addition to causing harm and devastation.

Obtaining radiological materials to combine with high explosives is not extremely difficult (at least for low-grade radiation material), but constructing the dirty bomb would be dangerous, as the radiation could burn and kill while the bomb was being assembled and transported.

Would-be attackers could find them too ineffective for their goals. For example, according to a United Nations report, Iraq tested a dirty-bomb device in 1987 but found that the radiation levels were too low to cause significant damage and so abandoned any further use of the device.

How Dangerous Is It?

While people could be killed by the blast itself, it is doubtful that the radioactivity produced after a dirty bomb would kill anyone. The radioactive material would be dispersed into the air and quickly reduced to low concentrations, thus only people within a few blocks of the explosion would be at risk of radiation exposure. In addition, because high-level radioactive materials from a nuclear facility are guarded and extremely difficult to obtain, it is much more likely that low-level sources would be used, such as might be found at hospitals, construction sites, and food-irradiation plants. The levels of radiation that would be created by the most probable sources would not be enough to cause severe illness from exposure.

Though it is possible that a low-level exposure of someone in the immediate vicinity might slightly increase the long-term risk of cancer, the risks are relatively minor. Doctors will be able to assess these risks after they determine the level of environmental exposure.

TIMELINE OF ILLNESS

Though most if not all injuries would be due to the explosion itself, the time to illness after radiation exposure depends on the radiation absorbed; symptoms may begin from minutes to weeks after a radiological incident. Exposure can continue to cause damage for years.

SYMPTOMS

The extent of radiation contamination depends on many factors, including the size of the explosive, the type and amount of radioactive material, weather conditions, the amount of radiation absorbed, the route of exposure, the length of time exposed, and the distance from the radiation source. Almost all deaths and serious injuries would probably be confined to the immediate vicinity of the explosion.

It is highly unlikely that symptoms of severe radiation exposure would occur after a dirty bomb. In fact, any material that could *cause* the severe exposure effects of acute radiation sickness (ARS) would be lethal in a matter of minutes to anyone transporting it in its pre-detonation form. Even a suicidal bomber would not be able to bring in enough radioactive material to create a significant radiation level after the explosion.

In the extremely unlikely event that someone was severely exposed to radiation, symptoms of RADIATION SICKNESS include upset stomach and vomiting; diarrhea; skin burns (redness, blistering); weakness, fatigue, exhaustion, fainting due to dehydration; inflammation of skin and mucous membranes (redness, tenderness, swelling, bleeding); hair loss; open sores in the mouth or along the intestinal tract; vomiting blood, bloody stool; bleeding from the nose, mouth, and gums; sloughing of skin; and open sores on the skin.

EMERGENCY RESPONSE

- **If you are potentially exposed to radiation, there are three basic ways to protect yourself:**
  1) Time. Decrease the time spent exposed to the radiation source.
  2) Distance. Get as far away from the source as possible.
  3) Shielding. Seek shelter, and create as thick a barrier as possible between you and the radiation. Even clothing and glass can shield from some types of radiation.
- **Cover your mouth and nose with fabric** (wet if possible) if in the immediate area.
- **The Centers for Disease Control recommends that you leave the immediate area** *by foot.* It you use public transportation, you may

spread contamination or become contaminated yourself by exposed people from the area. You could contaminate your own vehicle as well.

- **Shower as soon as possible with plenty of soap and change clothing** if you were in the immediate area and were potentially contaminated. Put exposed clothing in double plastic sealed bags. You may be advised to proceed to the nearest public monitoring and decontamination center.

- **Seek shelter at once** and remain until radiation levels have dropped if you are more than a few blocks away and not covered in residue. Go to a basement and/or inner room without windows if possible. If you are inside, remain inside.

- **Shut off ventilation systems** inside the shelter, including fans, air-conditioners, and forced-air heating units; close fireplace dampers.

- **Keep the radio or television on** to learn the determination of radiation involvement, and follow instructions provided by emergency officials.

- **Take potassium iodide** (see *TREATMENT* below) if instructed to do so.

- **Avoid potentially contaminated foods,** such as fruits and vegetables grown in the immediate area, until their safety has been determined.

- **Be prepared to evacuate.** Wearing hats or scarves, long-sleeved shirts, pants, and sturdy boots or shoes will offer some protection from radiological exposure.

- **If you are leaving the area,** determine which way the wind is blowing and go in the opposite direction (unless that is toward the blast site). Listen to local authorities for evacuation instructions.

TESTING AND DIAGNOSIS

Specialized equipment is required to determine the size of the affected area. Geiger counters can quickly measure radioactive contamination. They are available in more than 3,000 hospitals and are often carried by emergency personnel.

In most cases it is difficult to make a reliable estimate of radiation absorption in an individual. Samples of blood, urine, feces, vomit, and/or exposed metal clothing parts might be used to test the degree of exposure.

If a radioactive material was released, announcements will be made on television and radio as to where to report for radiation monitoring and tests to determine whether people were exposed to the radiation.

TREATMENT

Potassium iodide (KI) pills are effective in keeping the thyroid gland from absorbing radioactive iodine and thus may prevent thyroid cancer and other thyroid diseases from developing in the future. However, potassium iodide is not a universal radioactive remedy and would protect people only if radioactive iodine were released; it would be ineffective against other radioactive isotopes. Only nuclear fuel would release radioactive iodine, and the probability that it is the material in a dirty bomb is exceedingly small compared with the probability of it being lost or stolen medical or industrial sources. Further, keep in mind that only people in the immediate area of the explosion would be at risk for radiation poisoning.

The Centers for Disease Control states that because there is no way to know at the time of an incident whether radioactive iodine was used in the explosive device, and because potassium iodide can be dangerous to some people, taking potassium iodide is not recommended unless there is a known risk of exposure to radioactive iodine.

Adults over 40 years of age have the smallest risk of developing thyroid cancer or thyroid disease and a greater chance of having an allergic reaction, so potassium iodide is not recommended for adults over 40 unless they have been exposed to a very large dose of radioactive iodine.

Taking more potassium iodide than necessary offers no additional protection and can cause severe illness and death due to allergic reaction.

Listen for instructions from emergency officials as to whether you are in an area where you should take potassium iodide if the presence of radioactive iodine has been confirmed. If confirmed, one dose (130 mg) must be taken shortly before exposure or up to 3–4 hours after in order to be effective. One dose protects for 24 hours and is sufficient unless there is ongoing radiation. People should not take potassium iodide if they:

1) Have had thyroid disease,
2) Are allergic to iodine, and/or
3) Have certain skin disorders (e.g., dermatitis herpetiformis or urticarial vasculitis).

CHILDREN

- Children are at greater risk than adults of suffering damage from radiation exposure.
- Children 18 and under are at the greatest risk of developing thyroid cancer after exposure to radioactive iodine. Children over 1 month of age should ideally be given potassium iodide before radioactive iodine exposure or *as soon as possible* afterward. The recommended dose for children 3–18 years old is 65 mg; for children 1 month to 3 years, 32 mg; and for infants less than 1 month, 16 mg.

PREGNANCY

- Developing embryos and fetuses are particularly susceptible to radiation. Pregnant women should make every effort to avoid exposure and should be decontaminated immediately.

– Women who are breastfeeding and need to take potassium iodide should take the normal adult dosage.

SPECIAL PRECAUTIONS

Sometimes after a blast, a "secondary device" is used, meaning a second bomb is planted to detonate after an initial bomb goes off. These have been used to injure fleeing victims from the first attack or to harm emergency responders who arrive on the scene. Hence, do not assume that one explosion will be the last: when an explosion occurs, leave the area immediately.

ENVIRONMENTAL DECONTAMINATION AND CLEANUP

A dirty bomb blast would probably affect several city blocks. Although only low levels of radiation would be present, it could take weeks to months to decontaminate and be very costly.

HOW YOU CAN PREPARE

Keep health-facility and emergency phone numbers readily available (see *ADDITIONAL RESOURCES* below and the *Public Resources and Contact Information* section of the book).

Keep an evacuation kit prepared and ready to take with you (see Chapter 33, *Preparedness and Response Supplies*).

Keep potassium iodide pills on hand; know the risks and when to take them.

Gas masks, experts say, may help in protecting against particulate matter, since radiation attaches to particles in the air. However, when you get much beyond the area of the blast, the dust is going to dissipate quickly anyway. In addition, our medical experts do not recommend the use of gas masks except by those trained to use them because of the danger of improper use.

ADDITIONAL RESOURCES

Centers for Disease Control: Chemical/Biological/Radiological Hotline for obtaining information
    Hotline: 888-246-2675
Centers for Disease Control (CDC): Links to various radiological incident fact sheets
    www.cdc.gov/nceh/radiation/response.htm

Federal Emergency Management Agency (FEMA)
www.fema.gov
Phone: 800-480-2520, 202-646-4600

National Response Center: Chemical/Biological/Radiological Hotline for reporting incidents
Hotline: 800-424-8802

State public-health locator for officials, agencies, and public hotlines
www.statepublichealth.org

The Survival Guide: What to Do in a Biological, Chemical, or Nuclear Emergency website: For updates, supplementary information, and helpful links
www.911guide.com

U.S. Department of Energy: Radiation Emergency Assistance Center/Training Site
www.orau.gov/reacts
Phone: 865-576-1005

U.S. Nuclear Regulatory Commission
www.nrc.gov/reading-rm/doc-collections/fact-sheets/dirty-bombs.html
Radiation Protection Program: 301-415-8200

NUCLEAR BOMBS

RADIOACTIVE EVENT

Nuclear Bomb

DESCRIPTION

Massive explosion and radioactive fallout

TIME FROM EXPOSURE TO ILLNESS

Minutes to years

MAJOR SYMPTOMS

SEVERE EXPOSURE (radiation poisoning):
Burning of the skin with redness, blistering, and peeling; inflammation of skin and mucous membranes; dehydration; nausea; vomiting; diarrhea; convulsions; and exhaustion. Delayed symptoms include open sores on the skin and in the mouth or along the intestinal tract; gastrointestinal effects such as bloody diarrhea or stool and bloody vomit; bleeding from the nose, mouth, and gums; bruising; hair loss; and blindness

EMERGENCY RESPONSE

- Get as far away from the explosion site as quickly as possible; go against the wind unless that is toward the detonation site or you have been instructed to go a different direction by officials
- Cover your mouth and nose with a wet cloth
- Decontaminate as soon as you are away from the source of radiation
- Wash thoroughly with plenty of soap and water
- Shield yourself from the radiation source; use lead if possible
- Unless the building is in danger of collapsing, remain indoors and go to a basement if possible
- Turn off ventilation systems such as air-conditioning
- Listen to the radio or television for instructions from emergency management personnel
- Be prepared to evacuate
- Alternatively, you may be asked to shelter-in-place, possibly for 7 days or more

TREATMENT

Potassium iodide, chelating agents, nausea medication, probiotics, blood transfusion

POSSIBILITY OF DEATH

Depends upon distance from the explosion, duration of exposure, type of radiation, and route of exposure

WHAT IT IS

A nuclear bomb is the most destructive weapon known to man. "Nuclear bomb" and "nuclear weapon" are general terms that can refer to an ATOMIC, HYDRO-GEN, or NEUTRON BOMB (for a more detailed description, see Chapter 25, *Radiation Primer*). Nuclear explosions occur when masses of highly processed radioactive material are either suddenly thrust to-

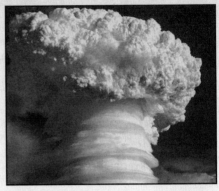

When a nuclear bomb explodes near the earth's surface, it pulls soil, matter, and water up into a mushroom cloud of radioactively contaminated dust and debris.

gether (fusion) or split apart (fission), triggering a violent chain reaction and release of energy. The explosion causes catastrophic damage to people, buildings, and the environment.

The bomb damage to man-made structures is due to two distinct causes: (1) a blast, or pressure wave, emanating from the center of the explosion, and (2) fires, caused either by the heat of the explosion itself or by the collapse of buildings containing flammable equipment and the like and the subsequent spread of those fires. Widespread radiation damage results when the bomb or missile explodes near the earth's surface and pulls soil, matter, and water up into a mushroom cloud, contaminating it with radiation. This radioactive matter, called fallout, settles back to the ground or is spread by the wind and is harmful to humans, causing acute illness or death or delayed reactions such as cancer years later.

WHAT IT DOES

The principal effects on the body from nuclear weapons are (1) blast, (2) thermal radiation, and (3) nuclear (ionizing) radiation. The ratio of effects depends upon the kind and size of the bomb; the approximate percentages below refer to atomic bombs.

1) A blast and pressure wave accounts for 50% of the energy released. The explosion creates a pressure wave that extends in all directions away from the blast, followed by a vacuum created by this wave. If the explosion occurs in the air, the pressure downward would destroy objects and people and the vacuum upward would produce the distinctive mushroom cloud of a nuclear detonation. An explosion on the ground would create a vast crater. Persons in the vicinity of the blast can be thrown due to the wave and then pulled back toward the blast by the vacuum, suffering injuries such as those sustained in a car accident. A large enough pressure wave would immediately disintegrate a human body. Lung tissue and gastrointestinal tissue are particularly susceptible to injury from this energy.

2) Thermal radiation (heat and light) accounts for 35% of the energy released. Once the bomb explodes, it releases an enormous fireball. This thermal radiation can cause burns in two ways—by direct absorption of heat through exposed surfaces (causing flash burns) or by secondary fires in the environment (flame burns). The bright flash from the initial fireball could cause eye injuries in the forms of temporary blindness, lasting 2–35 minutes (flash blindness), and permanent retinal scarring (only from directly viewing the fireball). The intense heat of raging fires would cause an updraft that would pull oxygen in and make it difficult to breathe in the surrounding area. In addition, as the lungs could be exposed to gases formed from indirect flames, lung injury would probably be common and would be responsible for high mortality rates.

3) Nuclear (ionizing) radiation accounts for 14% of the energy released (for a more detailed description of ionizing radiation, see Chapter 25, *Radiation Primer*). The initial ionizing radiation accounts for 4% and is composed of neutrons and gamma rays, the radioactive rays that are the most penetrating and harmful to humans. Residual ionizing radiation (fallout) accounts for the other 10% and comprises alpha particles (only harmful if ingested or inhaled), beta particles (which can cause skin injury), and gamma rays.

4) Electromagnetic pulse accounts for 1% of the energy released. Unique to a nuclear blast, the electromagnetic pulse is a massive surge of electrical power that is created the instant a nuclear detonation occurs and emanates from the center of the blast. It disables all electrical devices in its path, including anything with a computer chip. Note that this would pose an escape problem, as newer cars and other vehicles with computer chips would not be able to start.

Radiological Effects
Radiation kills or damages rapidly dividing cells such as blood-forming cells found in the bone marrow and cells that line the intestinal tract, which may lead to life-threatening dehydration and bone marrow failure. Disruption of normal cell functioning can sometimes lead to cancer many years later.

Nuclear Winter
Theoretically, if enough nuclear weapons were to go off, the resulting dust clouds from fallout and smoke from uncontrolled fires could block sunlight for several months, causing temperatures to drop below freezing. During

this "nuclear winter," plant life would die. Crops and farm animals, at least in the Northern Hemisphere, would be destroyed, and people would starve. In addition, the earth's ozone layer, which shields us from deadly solar ultraviolet radiation, would probably be hazardously damaged.

CAN YOU TELL IF YOU HAVE BEEN EXPOSED TO RADIOACTIVITY?

Radiological particles and materials are colorless, odorless, and tasteless and cannot be detected by humans without specialized equipment, such as a Geiger counter. The amount of radioactivity present after a blast would be highly variable, depending on the size and type of the bomb, your proximity, and weather conditions. Illness may not develop for weeks.

ASSESSMENT OF RISK

Risk of Use in an Attack

Risk of a nuclear bomb being built or stolen by terrorists: Building a large-scale nuclear weapon requires highly sophisticated technical skills and equipment, and detailed designs of these weapons remain secret. A greater concern is weapons such as "tactical nuclear weapons" falling into the hands of terrorists. These are mines, torpedoes, and short-range missiles with yields of 0.1 kiloton (which equals 100 tons of TNT) to up to 8 times the yield of the Hiroshima bomb. Many are small, making them vulnerable to theft, and even though they constitute a large percentage of the United States' and Russia's nuclear arsenals, they are the least-regulated category of nuclear weapons covered in arms-control agreements. However, because of the degree of complexity and difficulty of building or stealing one and the extraordinary amount of resources required in comparison to developing biological or chemical weapons, nuclear weapons are considered less likely to be utilized by terrorists than other methods.

Availability of nuclear fuel: The fuels to build the simplest, most reliable nuclear weapons are highly enriched uranium and plutonium, both of which are extremely expensive and heavily guarded. Uranium occurs naturally (there are between 1,300 and 2,100 metric tons in the world) but must be heavily processed to be weapons-grade. The uranium used in nuclear power plants is useless for bomb building. Plutonium does not occur in nature and can only be made in nuclear reactors; post–cold war, there may be about 100 tons left. The plutonium used in nuclear power plants could be used to make a bomb but would have to undergo a difficult and hazardous process of separating out the usable plutonium.

Governmental protection: Since September 11, 2001, the United States has increased funding for programs designed to keep radioactive materials out of terrorists' hands, including spending millions on increased security for Russia's weapons and nuclear materials. The United States has also increased its efforts and coordination with the CIA, FBI, and other intelligence agencies. In addition, the government has begun installing radiation detectors at airports, seaports, borders, railways, and highways around the country. Moreover, the newly developed Department of Homeland Security includes a division to address threats from weapons of mass destruction.

How Dangerous Is It?

Even a "small," 1-kiloton nuclear weapon—such as a crudely made or stolen weapon—would cause mass destruction and loss of life. For example, below is the damage a nuclear weapon might have upon the densely populated city of Manhattan:

	1 kiloton	150 kilotons
Initial Fatalities	200,000	800,000
Initial Injuries	200,000	900,000
Fallout	Could kill 50% of those as far as 3 miles away within a few weeks	Could kill 50% of those 10–15 miles away within a few weeks
Damage	Would demolish most buildings and other structures over 11 city blocks	Would demolish all buildings and structures within ½ mile of the blast site and spread fires that would burn out of control for days
Disruption	Would severely disrupt transportation, communications, utilities, and other infrastructure; emergency-response and medical facilities would be overwhelmed	Would knock out many of the city's major bridges and tunnels, as well as power grids, communication networks, and other crucial utilities such as water and gas, and destroy all but one of the city's major hospitals

(Council on Foreign Relations)

Radioactive fallout could cover an area of hundreds of miles. Large areas of land could be rendered useless because of persistent radioactivity in soil, water, and food. All living organisms in the vicinity could be affected immediately or for many years after exposure with the development of mutations and cancers. Long-term health, economic, psychological, political, and social consequences would likely be devastating for any American city. However, radiation is not as great a carcinogen as many people fear. People who survived the effects of radiation of a nuclear blast might only have an increased cancer risk of 15% (35% versus 20% baseline for unexposed people), as demonstrated by survivors of the Hiroshima and Nagasaki atomic bombs.

SYMPTOMS and TIMELINE OF ILLNESS

The symptoms and timeline of illness for radiation exposure can vary greatly with the amount and length of time of exposure and the total amount of radiation absorbed. Total radiation absorbed is measured in units of **sieverts (Sv)** (or rem, where 1 Sv = 100 rem). Scientists estimate that the average person in the United States receives a dose of about 3.33 millisieverts (1 millisievert = 1/1000 of a sievert) per year, which is equal to about 100 chest x-rays. If exposed to a dose greater than 2 Sv, a condition called acute radiation syndrome (ARS) develops. This is divided into four stages.

Acute Radiation Syndrome (ARS)

Stage 1: Symptoms begin with nausea and vomiting within minutes to hours after exposure and may last a few hours to a few days (usually the first 48–72 hours). Other symptoms of this stage may include diarrhea, intestinal cramps, salivation, dehydration, fatigue, weakness, apathy, fever, and low blood pressure.

Stage 2: A symptom-free phase begins hours to days after the beginning of symptoms and may last for 1–2½ weeks. The patient usually has no complaints during this stage, though blood cell populations are decreasing as a result of bone marrow damage. The greater the dose of radiation, the shorter this asymptomatic period will last.

Stage 3: This period begins in weeks 3–5 after exposure with severe abdominal pain, fever, bleeding, bruising, and infection. Each organ system may express its own symptoms depending on the amount of exposure.

    – *Central nervous system* (more than 15 Sv exposure). Sudden onset of fever, lethargy, loss of muscle control, altered mental status, tremors, seizures, and coma. Death can occur within several days.

    – *Cardiovascular system* (more than 15 Sv). Sudden onset of low blood pressure; irregular heartbeat due to death of heart tissue.

    – *Gastrointestinal system* (more than 5 Sv). Bloody diarrhea, nausea, vomiting, abdominal bloating, dehydration, and infection due to cell injury and death in the gastrointestinal lining.

    – *Hematopoietic syndrome* (more than 1–5 Sv). Total bone-marrow failure can occur, resulting in bruising, hemorrhage, and infection.

    – *Pulmonary syndrome* (more than 6–10 Sv). Inflammation of the lungs 1–3 months after exposure, which may lead to respiratory failure, lung scarring, and secondary damage to the heart months or years later.

Stage 4: The beginning of recovery may last weeks to months before illness resolves.

SKIN INJURY: In addition to initial skin burns from heat, people with ARS typically also have delayed skin damage due to the radiation. This damage can start to show within a few hours after exposure and can include swelling, itching, and redness (like a bad sunburn). As with other symptoms, the skin can heal for a short time before swelling, itching, and redness return. Complete healing can take from weeks to a few years, depending on the dose of radiation. There can also be hair loss.

EMERGENCY RESPONSE

- **If there is advanced warning of a nuclear-bomb attack in your area, your best response is to *EVACUATE*** in accordance with local authorities. Determine which way the wind is blowing, and go in the opposite direction if possible.

- **If there is a nuclear explosion, there are three basic ways to protect yourself:**
  1) Time. Decrease the time spent exposed to the radiation source.
  2) Distance. Get as far away from the source as possible.
  3) Shielding. Seek shelter, and create as thick a barrier as possible between you and the radiation. Even clothing and glass can shield from some types of radiation.

- **Do *not* look toward the site of detonation as it is happening,** as viewing the initial fireball could cause temporary blindness (which could be extremely dangerous in the immediate aftermath of the bomb) or permanent eye damage.

- **Be prepared to evacuate after a nuclear detonation.** Wearing hats or scarves, long-sleeved shirts, pants, and sturdy boots or shoes will offer some protection from radioactive fallout. Only specially designed protective wear for radioactivity can protect you from penetrating radiation in a highly contaminated area. Again, go in the direction against the wind (unless, of course, you would be going toward the detonation).

- **If you cannot evacuate, seek shelter at once** and remain there until radiation levels drop. Go to a basement without windows if possible. If you do not have a basement, go to an inner room without windows. You may be asked to shelter-in-place for several days (see *SPECIAL PRECAUTIONS* below).

- **Remove clothes and shoes** if you have been outside where fallout might have landed on you, and seal them in double plastic bags. Leave the bags outside before entering the shelter.

- **Shower thoroughly with plenty of soap.**

- **You may be advised to proceed to the nearest public monitoring and decontamination center.** No eating, drinking, or smoking would be allowed at these sites.

- **Shielding with lead** would be the most effective protection from the radioactive rays during and after an explosion.

- **Turn off ventilation systems** inside the shelter, including fans, air-conditioners, and forced-air heating units; close fireplace dampers.

- **Keep the radio or television on** and follow instructions provided by emergency management personnel, who may use the Emergency Broadcast System to disseminate important information to the public.

- **Avoid potentially contaminated foods,** such as fruits and vegetables grown in the area, until their safety has been determined.

- **Gas masks** help protect against inhalation of radioactive particles, which can cause internal contamination. However, the use of gas masks is not recommended to the untrained due to the danger of improper use.

- **Professional decontamination would include** chelating soap (known as green soap) and phosphate-based detergents (most detergents are) for external exposure, and chelating agents such as EDTA or DTPA, which bind to radioactive materials to remove them from the body, for internal decontamination. This regimen can remove up to 95% of radioactivity from an exposed individual. The water used to decontaminate would be collected and labeled as hazardous waste.

TESTING AND DIAGNOSIS

Specialized equipment is required to determine the size of the affected area. Geiger counters are used to measure radioactive contamination. They are available in more than 3,000 hospitals and are often carried by emergency personnel.

In most cases it is difficult to make a reliable estimate of radiation absorption in an individual. Samples of blood, urine, feces, vomit, and/or exposed metal clothing parts might be used to test the degree of exposure.

TREATMENT

Treatment may include **IV fluids** for hydration; **standard burn skin care**; **wounds gently washed** to prevent internal contamination; emergency management of nausea and vomiting with **antiemetics** (antinausea medicine); **management of pain** with morphine or acetaminophen (do not use aspirin, as it will interfere with blood clotting and make bleeding worse); **antibiotics** (recommended only if an infection takes hold); **blood**

transfusions; **blood-cell growth stimulants** if necessary for patients whose bone marrow is affected, which are most effective when given soon after exposure; **bone-marrow transplantation**, but it remains a controversial treatment; **probiotics**, which involve the use of bacterial implantation to recolonize the body's natural store of bacteria in the gastrointestinal tract, which we use to digest and absorb food; and **chelating agents** such as DTPA (the calcium form is used for early decontamination and the zinc form is used for long-term treatment).

Potassium Iodide (KI)

One dose of potassium iodide (130 mg)—available without a prescription at local pharmacies and over the Internet—is effective in keeping the thyroid gland from absorbing radioactive iodine and thus may prevent thyroid cancer from developing in the future. It protects for 24 hours. It must be taken shortly before exposure or up to 3–4 hours after in order to be effective. However, potassium iodide is not a universal radioactive remedy and protects people only if radioactive iodine has been released; it would be ineffective against other radioactive isotopes that may be present.

- People should not take potassium iodide if they:
  1) Have had thyroid disease,
  2) Are allergic to iodine, and/or
  3) Have certain skin disorders (e.g., dermatitis herpetiformis or urticarial vasculitis).

- Adults over 40 years of age have the smallest risk of developing thyroid cancer or thyroid disease and a greater chance of having an allergic reaction, so potassium iodide is not recommended for them unless they have been exposed to a very large dose of radioactive iodine.

- Taking more potassium iodide than necessary offers no additional protection and can cause severe illness and death due to allergic reaction.

- Listen for instructions from emergency officials as to whether you are in an area where you should take potassium iodide if the presence of radioactive iodine has been confirmed.

CHILDREN

- Children are at greater risk than adults of suffering damage from radiation exposure.

- Children 18 and under are at the greatest risk of developing thyroid cancer after exposure to radioactive iodine. Children over 1 month of age should ideally be given potassium iodide before radioactive iodine exposure or *as soon as possible* afterward. The recommended dose for children 3–18 years old is 65 mg, for children 1 month to 3 years, 32 mg, and for infants less than 1 month, 16 mg.

PREGNANCY

- Developing embryos and fetuses are particularly susceptible to radiation. Pregnant women should make every effort to avoid exposure and should be decontaminated immediately.
- Women who are breastfeeding and need to take potassium iodide should take the normal adult dosage.

SPECIAL PRECAUTIONS

People who live near but not in the immediate area of a nuclear attack may be asked to **shelter-in-place** rather than try to evacuate. Because many radioactive materials rapidly decay and dissipate, staying in your home may protect you from exposure to radiation. If you are outside when the alert is given, try to remove clothing and shoes, place them in sealed double plastic bags, and leave them outside before entering your shelter. The safest place in your home during a radioactive emergency is an inner room or the basement. The farther you are from windows, the safer you will be. Turn off any ventilation systems, close fireplace dampers, and seal windows, doors, and vents with duct tape; be sure to maintain enough ventilation to prevent suffocation. Keep water, food with a long shelf life, bedding, medicines, and anything else you may need for at least a 14-day stay in the shelter room (see Chapter 33, *Preparedness and Response Supplies*, for more suggestions on what to store). After 7 days the initial radioactivity will have decreased by 90%.

Note that the electromagnetic pulse following a nuclear bomb would disable computers for miles around, hence the Internet would not be useful for people within that vicinity. Phones, including cellular, would not work either. It is thus of utmost importance to have a family emergency plan to prepare for this event (see Chapter 30, *Creating an Emergency Action Plan*).

ENVIRONMENTAL DECONTAMINATION AND CLEANUP

Damage to the environment could last from decades to centuries, as water and soil are contaminated. Wind and flowing water can spread radiation over a wider area than the initial exposure.

Before contaminated areas could become habitable again, the government would have to reduce the radiation to a level strictly stipulated by the Environmental Protection Agency. Many areas would have to be evacuated and decontaminated, even if the actual health risk may not be that high. After a nuclear attack, radioactive materials would be physically lodged in crevices on the surfaces of buildings, sidewalks, streets, and so on, making the decontamination process very difficult. Some radioactive materials chemically bind with asphalt, concrete, and topsoil. It is so difficult to decontaminate, in fact, that much of the course of action may involve demolishing and removing contaminated buildings, roads, trees, plants, and soil and burying them under sand. Other methods used might be:

- Sandblasting contaminated surfaces, then washing and sealing them
- Chemically treating the soil and replanting new plants and trees to prevent winds from spreading contaminated dust and dirt
- Using certain types of fertilizer that absorb radiation to help reduce plant contamination

Water supplies in the immediate area could be contaminated from air fallout and water runoff. Radioactive sediments would settle on the bottom of bodies of water and in plants and fish living in the water.

HOW YOU CAN PREPARE

Keep an evacuation kit prepared and ready to take with you (see Chapter 33, *Preparedness and Response Supplies*).

Keep shelter-in-place supplies stocked (see *SPECIAL PRECAUTIONS* above and Chapter 33, *Preparedness and Response Supplies*) to last for at least 14 days.

Keep health-facility and emergency phone numbers readily available (see *ADDITIONAL RESOURCES* below and the *Public Resources and Contact Information* section of the book).

Know your community's emergency plan.

Have a family emergency plan that your whole family is aware of since phones and computers may not work after a nuclear detonation (see Chapter 30, *Creating an Emergency Action Plan*).

Electrical equipment may be protected by disconnecting it from its power source and placing it in or behind some type of shielding material.

Keep potassium iodide pills on hand.

Gas masks might help in protecting against particulate matter since radiation attaches to particles in the air. WARNING: Our medical experts do not recommend the use of gas masks except by those trained to use them. Data from Israel shows that the incorrect use of gas masks has caused many fatalities.

Know your blood type in case blood transfusions are necessary.

Fallout Shelters

Generally fallout shelters are below ground, are lined with concrete and steel, contain bedding, and are stocked with enough food, water, and other necessities for a 2-week stay. Ventilation and sanitation systems are installed in more sophisticated versions. It remains controversial how effective these structures would be in the event of a nuclear attack. Many experts maintain that evacuation remains the best course of action.

In the late 1950s and early 1960s the United States instituted a program of national fallout shelters and early-warning systems of sirens and emergency broadcasts. The fallout-shelter program was subsequently discontinued, and the signs for them (often yellow with a black radiation symbol) that remain today almost certainly do not lead to a functioning shelter.

ADDITIONAL RESOURCES

Centers for Disease Control (CDC): Chemical/Biological/Radiological
   Hotline for obtaining information: 888-246-2675
Centers for Disease Control: Links to various radiological fact sheets
   www.cdc.gov/nceh/radiation/response.htm
Center for Nonproliferation Studies
   www.cns.miis.edu
Council on Foreign Relations
   www.terrorismanswers.com
Federal Emergency Management Agency (FEMA)
   www.fema.gov
   Phone: 800-480-2520, 202-646-4600
National Response Center: Chemical/Biological/Radiological Hotline
   for reporting incidents: 800-424-8802
State public-health locator for officials, agencies, and public hotlines
   www.statepublichealth.org
The Survival Guide: What to Do in a Biological, Chemical, or Nuclear
   Emergency website: For updates, supplementary information, and
   helpful links
   www.911guide.com
U.S. Department of Energy: Radiation Emergency Assistance Center
   www.orau.gov/reacts
   Phone: 865-576-1005
U.S. Department of Homeland Security
   www.whitehouse.gov/deptofhomeland
World Health Organization (WHO): Radiation Emergency Medical
   Preparedness and Assistance Network (REMPAN)
   www.who.int/peh/radiation/rempan.html

NUCLEAR REACTORS

NUCLEAR WEAPONS

CHAPTER
28

RADIOACTIVE EVENT

Leak or Explosion at Nuclear Power Plant

DESCRIPTION

Radioactive exposure, environmental contamination

TIME FROM EXPOSURE TO ILLNESS

Minutes to years

MAJOR SYMPTOMS OF EXPOSURE

Though acute radiation poisoning after a nuclear reactor release is highly unlikely except for those in the immediate vicinity, symptoms of severe exposure include burning of the skin with redness, blistering, and peeling; inflammation of skin and mucous membranes; dehydration; nausea; vomiting; diarrhea; convulsions; and exhaustion. Delayed symptoms include open sores on the skin and in the mouth or along the intestinal tract; gastrointestinal effects such as bloody diarrhea or stool, bloody vomit; bleeding from the nose, mouth, and gums; bruising; and hair loss

EMERGENCY RESPONSE

— Get as far away as possible from the radiation source immediately; go against the wind unless that is toward the nuclear facility or you have been instructed to go a different direction by officials
— Cover your mouth and nose with a wet cloth
— Decontaminate as soon as you are away from the source of radiation
— Wash thoroughly with plenty of soap and water
— Shield yourself from the radiation source; use lead if possible
— Remain indoors and go to a basement without windows if possible or else an inner room
— Turn off ventilation systems such as air-conditioning
— Listen to the radio or television for instructions from emergency management personnel
— Be prepared to evacuate
— Alternatively, you may be asked to shelter-in-place, possibly for 7 days or more

TREATMENT

Potassium iodide, chelating agents, nausea medication, probiotics, blood transfusion

POSSIBILITY OF DEATH

Depends upon distance from the facility, duration of exposure, type of radiation, and route of exposure

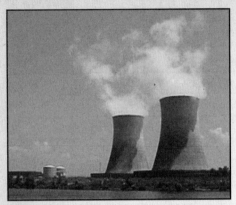

Seqoyah Nuclear Power Plant,
Tennessee

WHAT IT IS

Nuclear power plants use the process of nuclear fission to create energy. By splitting atoms in what is called a nuclear reactor, large amounts of energy are given off and if controlled can be harnessed to produce electricity (see Chapter 25, *Radiation Primer*, for a more detailed explanation). Nuclear reactors are also used in vessels such as submarines and ships, as nuclear power is particularly suitable for vessels that need to be at sea for long periods without refueling or for powerful submarine propulsion. In this chapter we will focus on nuclear power plants.

A nuclear plant cannot blow up like a nuclear bomb because a power plant does not keep its radioactive fuel (enriched uranium or plutonium) compact enough to set off the intense and rapid chain reaction needed for a bomb explosion. However, U.S. Homeland Security planners are worried about the following scenarios:

- Release of massive amounts of radiation after a nuclear plant is hit by a bomb (e.g., delivered by truck or boat)
- A large, commercial airliner made to crash into a nuclear facility
- Sabotage at a nuclear power plant by intruders or an insider

If any of these were to happen, large amounts of radiation could be released into the surrounding area.

The U.S. Nuclear Regulatory Commission currently licenses 104 nuclear power plants, which generate about 20% of our nation's electricity, as well as 36 non-power reactors at universities.

WHAT IT DOES

A meltdown or explosion at a nuclear facility could cause a large amount of radioactive material to be released and people in the surrounding area could be exposed or contaminated. Massive release of radiation could make an area uninhabitable for decades and even centuries.

Radiological Effects

Radiation kills or damages rapidly dividing cells such as blood-forming cells found in the bone marrow and cells that line the intestinal tract, which may lead to life-threatening dehydration and bone marrow failure. Disruption of normal cell functioning can sometimes lead to cancer many years later.

CAN YOU TELL IF YOU HAVE BEEN EXPOSED TO RADIOACTIVITY?

Radiological particles and materials are colorless, odorless, and tasteless and cannot be detected by humans without specialized equipment, such as a Geiger counter. The amount of radioactivity present after a power-plant explosion or leak would be highly variable, depending on the size and type of the incident, your proximity, and weather conditions. Illness may not develop for weeks.

ASSESSMENT OF RISK

Risk of Use in an Attack

In his January 2002 State of the Union address, President George W. Bush stated that among al-Qaeda materials U.S. forces found in Afghanistan were diagrams of American nuclear power plants and training manuals that listed nuclear power plants as among the best targets to spread fear in the United States. However, all U.S. nuclear power plants are heavily guarded by their own security systems and forces, which are supervised by the U.S. Nuclear Regulatory Commission (NRC). Further, their containment walls are made of concrete 2–5 feet thick with a steel lining, and they are designed to withstand things like earthquakes, tornadoes, hurricanes, and small plane crashes. The NRC has commissioned studies to determine what the impact of a large commercial airliner crash would be on such a facility. Some believe that because nuclear facilities are so well protected, terrorists might try other targets instead.

How Dangerous Is It?

Radioactive fallout could cover an area of hundreds of miles. Large tracts of land could be rendered useless because of persistent radioactivity in soil, water, and food. All living organisms in the vicinity could be effected immediately or for many years after exposure with the development of mutations and cancers. However, acute radiation sickness, as would be caused after a nuclear-bomb detonation, would likely only occur in first responders and to people working in the plant.

SYMPTOMS and TIMELINE OF ILLNESS

The symptoms and timeline of illness for radiation exposure can vary greatly with the amount and length of time of exposure and the total amount of radiation absorbed. Total radiation absorbed is measured in units of sieverts (Sv) (or rem, where 1 Sv = 100 rem). Scientists estimate that the average person in the United States receives a dose of about 3.33 millisieverts (1 millisievert = 1/1000 of a sievert) from natural exposure per year, which is equal to about 100 chest x-rays.

      If exposed to a dose greater than 2 Sv, a victim can develop a condition of severe radiation exposure called acute radiation syndrome (ARS). It is highly unlikely that a nuclear reactor leak or explosion would result in mass radiation poisoning casualties, as might occur after a nuclear bomb detonation. Severe radiation exposure would probably only involve first responders to the scene and the people who worked at the plant.

      In the unlikely event that someone was severely exposed to radiation, symptoms of ACUTE RADIATION SYNDROME include upset stomach and vomiting; diarrhea; skin burns (redness, blistering); weakness, fatigue, exhaustion, fainting due to dehydration; inflammation of skin and mucous membranes (redness, tenderness, swelling, bleeding); hair loss; open sores in the mouth or along the intestinal tract; vomiting blood; bloody stool; bleeding from the nose, mouth, and gums; sloughing of skin; and open sores on the skin. See Chapter 27, *Nuclear Bomb, SYMPTOMS*, for a more detailed description of the syndrome stages.

EMERGENCY RESPONSE

In the event of a terrorist attack on a nuclear power plant, a national emergency response that has been planned and rehearsed by local, state, and federal agencies for more than 20 years will be initiated. If you live near a nuclear power plant and have not received information that describes the emergency plan for that particular facility, contact the plant and ask for a copy of that information. You and your family should study the plan and be prepared to follow instructions from local and state public-health officials.

- **If there is advanced warning of a nuclear attack in your area, your best response is to** *EVACUATE* in accordance with local authorities. Determine which way the wind is blowing, and go in the opposite direction if possible.

- **If you are potentially exposed to radiation, there are three basic ways to protect yourself:**
  1) Time. Decrease the time spent exposed to the radiation source.

2) Distance. Get as far away from the source as possible.

3) Shielding. Seek shelter, and create as thick a barrier as possible between you and the radiation. Even clothing and glass can shield from some types of radiation.

- **Be prepared to evacuate.** Wearing hats or scarves, long-sleeved shirts, pants, and sturdy boots or shoes will offer some protection from radioactive fallout. Only specially designed protective wear for radioactivity can protect you from penetrating radiation in a highly contaminated area. Again, go in the direction against the wind (unless, of course, that is toward the power plant).

- **If you cannot evacuate, seek shelter at once** and remain there until radiation levels drop. Go to a basement without windows if possible. If you do not have a basement go to an inner room without windows. You may be asked to shelter-in-place for several days (see *SPECIAL PRECAUTIONS* below). After 7 days, radioactivity would be only 10% of initial levels.

- **Remove clothes and shoes,** seal in double plastic bags, and leave outside before entering shelter if possible.

- **Shower thoroughly with plenty of soap.**

- **You may be advised to proceed to the nearest public monitoring and decontamination center.** No eating, drinking, or smoking would be allowed at these sites.

- **Shielding with lead** would be the most effective protection from the radioactive rays during and after an explosion.

- **Turn off ventilation systems** inside the shelter, including fans, air-conditioners, and forced-air heating units; close fireplace dampers.

- **Keep the radio or television on** and follow instructions provided by emergency management personnel, who may use the Emergency Broadcast System to disseminate important information to the public.

- **Avoid potentially contaminated foods,** such as fruits and vegetables grown in the surrounding area, until their safety has been determined.

- **Don't panic.** Evacuation and decontamination after low-level radiological contamination can be delayed for days or weeks without serious health effects.

- **Gas masks** may help in protecting against inhalation of radioactive particles, which can cause internal contamination. However, the use of gas masks is not recommended to the untrained due to the danger from improper use. Alternatively, cover your mouth with a wet cloth.

- **Professional decontamination would include** chelating soap (known as green soap) and phosphate-based detergents (most detergents are) for external exposure, and chelating agents such as EDTA or DTPA, which bind to radioactive materials to remove them from the body, for internal decontamination. This regimen can remove up to 95% of radioactivity from an exposed individual. The water used to decontaminate would be collected and labeled as hazardous waste.

TESTING AND DIAGNOSIS

Specialized equipment is required to determine the size of the affected area. Geiger counters are used to measure radioactive contamination. They are available in more than 3,000 hospitals and are often carried by emergency personnel.

In most cases it is difficult to make a reliable estimate of radiation absorption in an individual. Samples of blood, urine, feces, vomit, and/or exposed metal clothing parts might be used to test the degree of exposure.

TREATMENT

Many of the following treatments apply only for severe radiation exposure, which would only occur to those in the immediate vicinity of the nuclear reactor: **IV fluids** for hydration; **standard burn skin care**; **antiemetics** (anti-nausea medicine) to control nausea and vomiting; **pain management** with morphine or acetaminophen (do not use aspirin as it will interfere with blood clotting and make bleeding worse); **antibiotics** if an infection takes hold; **blood transfusions**; **blood-cell growth stimulants** if bone marrow is affected (these are most effective when given soon after exposure); **bone marrow transplantation** (a controversial treatment); **probiotics** (implanting bacteria to recolonize the body's natural store of bacteria in the gastrointestinal tract, which we use to digest and absorb food), and **chelating agents** such as DTPA (the calcium form is used for early decontamination and the zinc form for long-term treatment).

Potassium Iodide (KI)

One dose of potassium iodide (130 mg)—available without a prescription at local pharmacies and over the Internet—is effective in keeping the thyroid gland from absorbing radioactive iodine and thus may prevent thyroid cancer from developing in the future. It protects for 24 hours and should not need to be taken again if there is no ongoing radiation. It must be taken shortly before exposure or up to 3–4 hours after in order to be effective. However, potassium iodide is not a universal radioactive remedy and protects people only if radioactive iodine has been released; it is ineffective against other radioactive isotopes that may be present.

- People should not take potassium iodide if they:
  1) Have had thyroid disease,
  2) Are allergic to iodine, and/or
  3) Have certain skin disorders (e.g., dermatitis herpetiformis or urticarial vasculitis).
- Adults over 40 years of age have the smallest risk of developing thyroid cancer or thyroid disease and a greater chance of having an allergic reaction, so potassium iodide is not recommended for them unless they have been exposed to a very large dose of radioactive iodine.
- Taking more potassium iodide than necessary offers no additional protection and can cause severe illness and death due to allergic reaction.
- Listen for instructions from emergency officials as to whether you are in an area where you should take potassium iodide if the presence of radioactive iodine has been confirmed.

CHILDREN

- Children are at greater risk than adults of suffering damage from radiation exposure.
- Children 18 and under are at the greatest risk of developing thyroid cancer after exposure to radioactive iodine. Children over 1 month of age should ideally be given potassium iodide before radioactive iodine exposure or *as soon as possible* afterward. The recommended dose for children 3–18 years old is 65 mg; for children 1 month to 3 years, 32 mg; and for infants less than 1 month, 16 mg.

PREGNANCY

- Developing embryos and fetuses are particularly susceptible to radiation. Pregnant women should make every effort to avoid exposure and should be decontaminated immediately.
- Women who are breastfeeding and need to take potassium iodide should take the normal adult dosage.

SPECIAL PRECAUTIONS

People who live near but not in the immediate area of a nuclear facility may be asked to **shelter-in-place** rather than try to evacuate. Because many radioactive materials rapidly decay and dissipate, staying in your home may protect you from exposure to radiation. If you are outside when the alert is given, try to remove clothing and shoes, place them in sealed double plastic bags, and leave them outside before entering your shelter. The safest place in your home during a radioactive emergency is an inner room or the basement. The farther you are from windows, the safer you will be. Turn off any ventilation systems, close fireplace dampers, and seal windows, doors, and vents with duct tape; be sure to maintain enough ventilation to prevent suffocation. Keep water, food with a long shelf life, bedding, medicines, and anything else you may need for at least a 7-day stay in the shelter room (see Chapter 33, *Preparedness and Response Supplies*, for more suggestions on what to store). After 7 days the initial radioactivity will have decreased by 90%.

If you must go outside for critical or lifesaving activities, cover your nose and mouth with a wet cloth and avoid stirring up and breathing any dust. Remember that going outside could increase your exposure and possibly spread contamination to others.

Be aware that trained monitoring teams will be moving through areas of potential radiation exposure wearing special protective clothing and equipment to determine the extent of possible contamination. These teams will wear protective gear as a precaution and not as an indication of the risks to those in the area.

ENVIRONMENTAL DECONTAMINATION AND CLEANUP

Damage to the surrounding environment could last from decades to centuries, as water and soil are contaminated. Wind and flowing water can spread radiation over a wider area than the initial exposure.

Before contaminated areas become habitable, the government would have to reduce the radiation to a level strictly stipulated by the Environmental Protection Agency. Many areas would have to be evacuated and decontaminated, even if the actual health risk may not be that high. After radioactive fallout, radioactive materials would be physically lodged in crevices on the surfaces of buildings, sidewalks, streets, and so on, making the decontamination process very difficult. Some radioactive materials chemically bind with asphalt, concrete, and topsoil. It is so difficult to decontaminate, in fact, that the course of action may involve demolishing and removing contaminated buildings, roads, trees, plants, and soil and burying them under sand. Other methods used might be:

- Sandblasting contaminated surfaces, then washing and sealing them
- Chemically treating the soil and planting new plants and trees to prevent winds from spreading contaminated dust and dirt
- Using certain types of fertilizer that absorb radiation to help reduce plant contamination

Water supplies in the immediate area could be contaminated from air fallout and water runoff. Radioactive sediments would settle on the bottom of bodies of water and in plants and fish living in the water.

HOW YOU CAN PREPARE

Keep an evacuation kit prepared and ready to take with you (see Chapter 33, *Preparedness and Response Supplies*).

Keep shelter-in-place supplies stocked (see *SPECIAL PRECAUTIONS* above and Chapter 33, *Preparedness and Response Supplies*) to last for at least 7 days.

Keep health-facility and emergency phone numbers readily available (see *ADDITIONAL RESOURCES* below and the *Public Resources and Contact Information* section of the book).

Your community should have a plan in case of a radiation emergency that is coordinated with local and federal officials and any nearby nuclear facilities. Check with community leaders to learn more about the plan and possible evacuation routes.

Check with your child's school, the nursing home of a family member, and your employer to see what their plans are for dealing with a radiation emergency.

Have a family emergency plan that your whole family is aware of (see Chapter 30, *Creating an Emergency Action Plan*).

Keep potassium iodide pills on hand.

Gas masks might help in protecting against particulate matter since radiation attaches to particles in the air. WARNING: Our medical experts do not recommend the use of gas masks except by those trained to use them. Data from Israel shows that the incorrect use of gas masks has caused many fatalities.

Know your blood type in case blood transfusions are necessary.

Fallout Shelters

Generally fallout shelters are below ground, are lined with concrete and steel, contain bedding, and are stocked with enough food, water, and other necessities for a 2-week stay. Ventilation and sanitation systems are installed in more sophisticated versions. It remains controversial how effective these structures would be in the event of nuclear fallout. Many experts maintain that evacuation remains the best course of action.

In the late 1950s and early 1960s the United States instituted a program of national fallout shelters and early-warning systems of sirens and emergency broadcasts. The fall-out shelter program was subsequently discontinued, and the signs for them (often yellow with a black radiation symbol) that remain today almost certainly do not lead to a functioning shelter.

ADDITIONAL RESOURCES

Centers for Disease Control (CDC): Links to various radiological incident fact sheets
www.cdc.gov/nceh/radiation/response.htm

Centers for Disease Control: Chemical/Biological/Radiological Hotline for obtaining information
Hotline: 888-246-2675

Council on Foreign Relations
www.terrorismanswers.com

Federal Emergency Management Agency (FEMA)
www.fema.gov
Phone: 800-480-2520, 202-646-4600

International Nuclear Safety Center (operated by Argonne National Laboratory for the U.S. Department of Energy): Locations of nuclear power reactors in the United States
www.insc.anl.gov/pwrmaps/map/united_states.php

National Response Center: Chemical/Biological/Radiological Hotline for reporting incidents
Hotline: 800-424-8802

State public-health locator for officials, agencies, and public hotlines
www.statepublichealth.org

The Survival Guide: What to Do in a Biological, Chemical, or Nuclear Emergency website: *www.911guide.com*

U.S. Department of Energy
www.energy.gov
Phone: 800-DIAL-DOE (800-342-5363)

U.S. Department of Energy: Radiation Emergency Assistance Center
www.orau.gov/reacts
Phone: 865-576-1005

U.S. Environmental Protection Agency (EPA)/Radiological Emergency Response: Counter-terrorism and links to Chemical Emergency Preparedness and Prevention
www.epa.gov/radiation/rert/ct.htm

U.S. Nuclear Regulatory Commission
www.nrc.gov/reactors.html

World Health Organization (WHO): Radiation Emergency Medical Preparedness and Assistance Network (REMPAN)
www.who.int/peh/Radiation/rempan.html

EVENT WITH UNKNOWN RADIOACTIVITY

EVENT

Event in which the presence of radioactivity is undetermined

DESCRIPTION

Bomb, explosion, airborne release, leak, fallout

POSSIBLE EARLY SYMPTOMS

Symptoms of severe radiation exposure (which would likely only occur after a nuclear bomb or to people very short distances from radiation source): Nausea, vomiting, skin reddening, diarrhea, intestinal cramps, salivation, dehydration, fatigue, weakness, apathy, fever, and low blood pressure

EMERGENCY RESPONSE

- Get as far away from the potential radiation source as possible immediately, going against the wind unless instructed otherwise
- Cover your mouth and nose with fabric (wet if possible) if in the immediate area
- If the building is not in danger of collapsing, remain there and go to a basement without windows if possible or else an inner room
- If outside and in the vicinity, seek shelter
- Shield yourself from the potential radiation source; use lead if possible
- Wash thoroughly with soap and water as soon as you are away from the potential source of radiation
- Turn off ventilation systems such as air-conditioning
- Listen to television or radio for instructions from emergency management personnel
- Be prepared to evacuate
- Alternatively, you may be asked to shelter-in-place for several days

TREATMENT

Once radiation exposure confirmed: potassium iodide, chelating agents, nausea medication, probiotics, blood transfusion

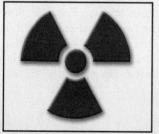

The radiation symbol was first created at a University of California at Berkeley radiation lab in 1946. It is used today to signify the presence or potential use of radioactivity. Signs with this symbol indicating nuclear-fallout shelters are remnants of the 1950s and 1960s—the shelters they were intending to identify almost certainly no longer exist.

OVERVIEW

Radiological materials are colorless, odorless, and tasteless and cannot be detected without specialized equipment. In addition, symptoms can be delayed for weeks or years. Hence, when there is a potential radiological emergency, until it is confirmed by public-health officials that there is no risk of contamination, presume you may be exposed to radiation. Three scenarios in which this might are occur are (1) a DIRTY BOMB explosion (see Chapter 26), (2) dispersal of radioactive substances without the use of explosives, such as by airborne release, and (3) a NUCLEAR POWER PLANT breach or explosion (see Chapter 28). If you are in the area of these incidents, take the necessary precautions (see table above, *Emergency Response*). Because the determination of radiation dispersal will probably be made rapidly, we have not gone into great detail in terms of response in this chapter. It is important to keep apprised of emergency-official broadcasts for confirmation of radioactivity after a suspected event.

NATIONAL, STATE, AND LOCAL RESPONSES TO AN ATTACK

State and local authorities have the primary responsibility of responding to a radiation attack. There are emergency management offices in all 50 states, with response plans tailored to local situations. The Metropolitan Medical Response System (MMRS) coordinates emergency response in major U.S. cities (around 120 so far) involving weapons of mass destruction, including dirty bombs.

Federal agencies are organized to help state and local authorities respond. The U.S. Department of Energy maintains the Nuclear Emergency Search Team to respond to threats of nuclear and radiological attacks within the United States. After a nuclear explosion, the Federal Emergency Management Agency (FEMA) would coordinate with the Environmental Protection Agency (EPA), the FBI, and the Departments of Energy, Defense, and Homeland Security. The EPA has a radiological emergency response team composed of scientists, doctors, engineers, and agents with special training and equipment that can be dispatched to anywhere in the country. The U.S. Department of Health and Human Services has purchased 1.6 million doses—and plans to purchase 5–10 million more—of potassium iodide in the event of emergency radioactive iodine exposure, such as might occur after a nuclear bomb or nuclear reactor explosion. The federal government would also provide long-term support, assistance, and resources to state and local disaster efforts.

In the event of a terrorist attack on a nuclear power plant, a national emergency response plan that includes local, state, and federal agencies would be initiated. The plants themselves are required by the U.S. Nuclear Regulatory Commission to have extensive, detailed safety and emergency plans. If you live near a nuclear power plant and have not received information that describes the emergency plan for that particular facility, contact the plant and ask for a copy of that information.

INDICATORS OF A POSSIBLE RADIOLOGICAL INCIDENT

Radiation is undetectable by humans without specialized equipment, such as a Geiger counter.

Unusual numbers of sick or dying people and/ or animals	A large number of casualties could indicate a radiological incident has taken place. The time before symptoms are observed depends upon the radioactive material used and the dose received, so it is highly variable (minutes to weeks)
Unusual metal debris	Unexplained bomb/munitions-like material
Radiation symbols	Containers may display a radiation symbol (see image above)
Heat-emitting material	Material that seems to emit heat without any sign of an external heating source
Glowing material/particles	If the material is strongly radioactive, it may emit a radioluminescence
Aerosolized solid or liquid	Airborne substance release, such as by crop duster

(From *"Chemical/Biological/Radiological Incident Handbook,"* by the Chemical, Biological and Radiological (CBRN) Subcommittee, 1998.)

EMERGENCY RESPONSE

If you are exposed to radiation, there are three basic ways to protect yourself:

    1) Time. Decrease the time spent exposed to the radiation source.

    2) Distance. Get as far away from the source as possible.

    3) Shielding. Seek shelter, and create as thick a barrier as possible between you and the radiation. Even clothing and glass can shield from some types of radiation.

If a radiation incident is confirmed, follow the detailed emergency-response section of the respective chapter (Chapter 26, *Dirty Bombs;* Chapter 27, *Nuclear Bombs;* Chapter 28, *Nuclear Reactors*). In the event of an aerosol release of a potentially radioactive substance, follow the emergency response recommendations for dirty bombs, with the exception that you should rinse off with copious amounts of water as soon as possible (shower with soap if possible).

SPECIAL PRECAUTIONS

Be aware that trained monitoring teams will be moving through areas of potential radiation exposure wearing special protective clothing and equipment to determine the extent of possible contamination. These teams will wear protective gear as a precaution and not as an indication of the risks to those in the area.

The possibility of exposure to radiation may elicit short- and long-term fear and stress reactions. Common acute stress reactions include insomnia, impaired concentration, and even social withdrawal. Since several psychological symptoms mimic those of radiation exposure such as nausea, vomiting, and rash, exposure cannot be confirmed by clinical symptoms alone. Groups at high risk for psychological effects include children, pregnant women, mothers of young children, emergency and cleanup workers, and persons with a history of mental illness. If you or someone you know has trouble coping, do not hesitate to seek help from a mental health specialist.

ADDITIONAL RESOURCES

American Psychological Association
  helping.apa.org/daily/terrorism.html
Centers for Disease Control (CDC): Links to radiological fact sheets
  www.cdc.gov/nceh/radiation/response.htm
Centers for Disease Control: Chemical/Biological/Radiological Hotline
  for obtaining information: 888-246-2675
Federal Emergency Management Agency (FEMA)
  www.fema.gov
  Phone: 800-480-2520, 202-646-4600
Metropolitan Medical Response System (MMRS)
  www.mmrs.hhs.gov
National Response Center: Chemical/Biological/Radiological Hotline
  for reporting incidents: 800-424-8802
State public-health locator for officials, agencies, and public hotlines
  www.statepublichealth.org
U.S. Department of Energy
  www.energy.com
U.S. Nuclear Regulatory Commission
  www.nrc.gov/reading-rm/doc-collections/fact-sheets/dirty-bombs.html

CREATING AN EMERGENCY ACTION PLAN

Almost any one of the scenarios described in this book could occur quickly and without warning, forcing you to evacuate your neighborhood or confining you to your home. Because communication with your family members and loved ones may be impossible during an event, it is imperative that you and your family design an emergency plan and commit it to memory.

EMERGENCY PLAN

- **Discuss with your children the kinds of emergencies that are likely to occur** and for which they should be prepared.
- **Find out about the disaster plans** for your workplace, your children's schools and day care center, and other places where your family spends time.
- **Learn about your community's warning signals**—what they mean and what you should do when you hear them.
- **Assemble an *evacuation kit*** (see Chapter 33, *Preparedness and Response Supplies*).
- **Assemble *shelter-in-place supplies*** (see Chapter 33, *Preparedness and Response Supplies*).
- **Learn what to do in an evacuation** in your community. Discuss with family members.
- **Pick two places to meet in the event of an evacuation:**
  1. A place right outside your home in case of a sudden emergency in your home
  2. A place outside of your neighborhood in case you cannot return home
  Everyone should know the addresses and phone numbers of these places.
- **Agree upon an out-of-state friend or family member** who can be your family contact in the event of a large emergency and have that number with you at all times. After a disaster, it is often easier to get a long-distance call through than a local one, so this person can relay messages for you.
- **Remember that E-mail can sometimes get through when calls won't.**
- **Obtain your community's nuclear-emergency and evacuation plan.** If you live within 30 miles of a nuclear power plant, there should be a detailed response plan available to community residents. Contact the plant directly.

EVACUATION

- If local authorities have asked you to leave your home, they probably have a good reason.
- Bring an evacuation kit with you (see Chapter 33, *Preparedness and Response Supplies*).
- Follow travel routes that local authorities specify. Do not use shortcuts, as certain areas may be impassable or dangerous.
- If you have time, call your family contact to report where you will be going.

SOURCES FOR FOOD AND WATER IF NOT STORED FOR AN EMERGENCY

Food Sources

Bring canned food and other sealed, nonperishable foods into your shelter area. Do not bring in fresh fruits or vegetables from outside if there is potential airborne contamination. Try to prepare beforehand, as most cities have only a 5-day food supply or less.

If activity is reduced, healthy people can survive on half their usual food intake for an extended period and without any food for many days. Food, unlike water, may be rationed safely, except for children and pregnant women.

Water Sources

- Fill up bathtubs at the beginning of the emergency (water supplies could become contaminated later)
- Hot-water tanks and pipes
- Ice cubes
- Moving water such as streams, rivers, and rain. Pond or lake water if clear. Avoid water with floating material, an odor, or a dark color
- Water in the reservoir tanks of toilets (not the bowls), as a last resort

If water is not pure, you can strain large particles through paper towels, then treat it by one of the following methods:
1. Boil for 3–5 minutes.
2. Disinfect with 16 drops of household liquid bleach per gallon water, then let stand for 15–30 minutes.

ADDITIONAL RESOURCES

American Red Cross
www.redcross.org/services/disaster/beprepared/hsas.html
U.S. Department of Homeland Security: See link to Citizen Preparedness Guide
www.whitehouse.gov/homeland

CHILDREN

OVERVIEW

The chapters in this book devoted to biological, chemical, and nuclear weapons address specific precautions for children for those particular threats. This chapter addresses some general concerns, recommendations, and precautions for children, particularly in relation to emergency planning and coping with terrorism. Many of the recommendations here were adapted from resources developed by the American Academy of Pediatrics and the American Red Cross (see *ADDITIONAL RESOURCES* section below).

As the latter half of the chapter describes—because children are more vulnerable to most biological, chemical, and radiological weapons releases than adults—it is crucial to be highly vigilant about prevention, protection, and response strategies for them. Terrorists might even target children, as they did in 1995 when the FBI uncovered a plot to release a chlorine gas bomb in Disneyland.

Greater Vulnerability
- Infants, toddlers, and young children do not have the developed motor skills needed to escape from the site of a biological, chemical, or radiological emergency, nor do they have the cognitive ability to decide in which direction to flee.
- All children are at risk of psychological injury such as post-traumatic stress syndrome from experiencing or living through the threat of a biological, chemical, or nuclear terrorist event.
- Children are difficult to care for by persons wearing protective equipment, which is essential in the management of biological, chemical, and radiological emergencies.

EMERGENCY PLANNING

- **Discuss with your children the kinds of emergencies that are likely to occur** and for which they should be prepared. Make sure they know where to go in your home to stay safe.
- **Teach your child how to recognize danger signals,** such as community warning systems.
- **Explain to children how and when to call for help.** Keep emergency phone numbers (911 and other local emergency phone numbers) where every family member can find them.

- **Have children who are old enough memorize important family information,** including their full name, parents' names, address, and phone number.
- **Give each family member an emergency list** with the phone number of a family contact out of state (in case local phone lines are jammed) and the name, address, and phone number of an area meeting place in case of an evacuation.
- **Teach children how to reverse telephone charges** in order to make a call from a public telephone without change.
- **Find out about the disaster plans** for your children's school and day care center, and other places where they spend time.
- **Remember that some officials say schools may be the safest place for children.** The Red Cross recommends that if protective actions are being taken at your children's school (including sheltering-in-place or evacuating), you should not go to the school or call. You could tie up a phone line that is needed for emergency communications. For further information, listen to local emergency radio and TV stations to learn when and where you can pick up your children.
- **Consult your child's school regarding their policy for authorizing pickups** by someone other than the parents.
- **Include special items for infants and children in your *evacuation kit*** (see Chapter 33, *Preparedness and Response Supplies*), such as medications, formula, diapers, and entertainment.
- **Include special items for infants and children in your *shelter-in-place supplies*** (see Chapter 33, *Preparedness and Response Supplies*). Make sure your children know where the supplies are kept in the house.
- **Discuss with all family members what to do in an evacuation** in your community.

WHAT TO TELL CHILDREN / HELPING THEM COPE

A disaster may strike quickly and without warning. Such an event can be frightening for adults, but it is traumatic for children if they don't know what to do and are not helped through it emotionally. During a biological, chemical, or nuclear emergency, your family may have to leave your home and daily routine, and children may be aware of mass casualties. They may become anxious, confused, or frightened. It is important to give children guidance that will help reduce their fears.

What to Tell Your Children About Disasters and Terrorist Events
It is important to warn children, without overly alarming them, about disasters. Tell them that a disaster is something that could hurt people or cause damage. Talk about things that could happen at a level appropriate for their age; avoid graphic details. Tell children that there are many people

who can help them during a disaster so that they will not be afraid of firefighters, police officers, paramedics, or other emergency officials.

The American Academy of Pediatrics recommends explaining that terrorist acts are ones of desperation and horror—that there are "bad" people out there, and bad people do bad things, but not all people in a particular group are bad. If a group that carried out a terrorist incident is identified, children should know that lashing out at members of the group, such as a particular religious or ethnic group, will only cause more harm.

Reassure your children that there are lots of people working to keep them safe.

During a Biological, Chemical, or Nuclear Emergency

- One of the most important things a parent can do for a child in an emergency situation is to stay calm. Children of all ages can easily pick up on their parents' fears and anxieties. In a disaster, they'll look to their parents for clues on how to act. If you react with alarm, the child may become more scared. They see fear in adults as proof that the danger is real.
- No matter how old the child, be honest and start with basic facts, using simple, direct language to describe what is going on. They don't need to know everything; base the amount of information and level of detail on what's appropriate for their age. Graphic details are not necessary and should be avoided.
- Explain what will be happening next. For example, say, "Tonight we will all stay together in the shelter." Get down and speak at your child's eye level.
- Children depend on daily routines: they wake up, eat breakfast, go to school, play with friends. Recognize that when emergencies or disasters interrupt this routine, they may become anxious.
- Limit television broadcasts, and when children watch, watch with them. Keep in mind that very young children may believe the event is happening over and over again each time they see it broadcast.
- Children's fears may stem from their imagination, and you should take these feelings seriously. Your words and actions can provide reassurance.

After a Biological, Chemical, or Nuclear Emergency

- Take care of yourself first. Children depend on the adults around them to make them feel safe and secure. If you are very anxious or angry, children are likely to be more affected by your emotional state than your words.
- Immediately after the event, try to reduce your child's fear and anxiety. Your response during this time may have a lasting impact. Be aware that after a disaster, children are most afraid that:
  • The event will happen again.
  • Someone will be injured or killed.

- They will be separated from the family.
- They will be left alone.

- Reassure children of the steps that are being taken to keep them safe.
- Try to keep the family together as much as possible. Children get anxious and worry that their parents will never return.
- Let children participate in the family's recovery activities. Giving them chores that are their responsibility will help them feel that their life will return to normal and that everything will be all right.
- Once the danger has passed, concentrate on your children's emotional needs by asking them what is uppermost in their mind. To not talk about it makes the event seem even more threatening, so encourage your children to talk about the event and to ask as many questions as they want. Like adults, children are better able to cope with a crisis if they understand it. Encourage them to describe what they're feeling and listen to what they say. You could also encourage children to draw or paint pictures to describe how they are feeling about their experiences.
- Children may undergo a personality change after a traumatic event. They may regress in their social skills or revert to younger behavior such as bedwetting. A quiet, caring, obedient child might become selfish, noisy, and aggressive, or an outgoing child might become shy and afraid. They may have nightmares or not want their parents to leave their sight. Watch for unusual behavior. Some children may not show evidence of being upset for several weeks or even months.
- Older children and adolescents may not want to talk about it. Don't force them; just occasionally extend the invitation and wait until they are ready. Sometimes asking them what others are thinking about makes it easier for them to talk.
- You can help children cope by understanding what causes their anxieties and fears. Reassure them with firmness and love. Your children will realize that life will eventually return to normal. If a child does not respond to the above suggestions, seek help from a mental health specialist or a member of the clergy.

BIOLOGICAL EMERGENCIES
Greater Vulnerability
- Children are more likely to have minor scrapes and wounds, making it easier for bacteria, viruses, and toxins to enter the bloodstream.
- Many of the biological agents cause diarrhea and/or vomiting, and children are more likely to become severely dehydrated from it, which could lead to shock.
- Many vaccines and medications have not been studied in children as well as they have been in adults. Of available vaccines and drugs, not all are safe for young children.

- Children are often more susceptible to illnesses caused by biological agents than are adults because their immune systems are not fully developed yet.
- Because children breathe faster than adults, they would be exposed to relatively greater dosages of aerosolized biological agents.
- For all of these reasons, in the event of a suspected exposure to a biological contaminant, parents should take extra care to decontaminate their children and their surroundings, to seek medical care, and to monitor them for any signs of developing illness (especially fever, cough, rash, sluggishness, and difficulty breathing).

Infection Prevention
To protect your child against catching something while at school or day care, the College of American Pathologists offers the following recommendations:
- Make sure that the staff at your child's school has been trained to use prevention techniques and practices them regularly.
- Staff should ask the children who are old enough to wash their hands during the day, especially before eating and after using the bathroom. Hands should be washed thoroughly; having children say their ABCs while they wash should ensure they spend enough time on the task.
- Staff should wash their own hands frequently, use disposable towels, change diapers in a special place, wash toys frequently, and assign food service to a single person. These infection-control policies have been shown to work in hospitals and nursing homes as well as day care centers, so don't be afraid to insist on them.

Special Precautions
The following are some of the antibiotics that have special precautions for infants and children: chloramphenicol, ciprofloxacin, doxycycline, streptomycin, tetracycline, and trimethoprim-sulfamethoxazole (Bactrim).

CHEMICAL EMERGENCIES
Greater Vulnerability
- Because many of the chemicals that might be used in a terrorist attack are heavier than air, children might be disproportionately affected merely because they are closer to the ground.
- Because children breathe faster than adults, they would be exposed to relatively greater dosages of aerosolized chemical agents.
- For their body weight, children have a greater skin surface area than adults, which could expose them more to chemical substances that affect the skin, such as blister agents. In addition, the skin of newborns and children is more permeable, which would make agents that are absorbed through the skin more dangerous.

NUCLEAR / RADIOLOGICAL EMERGENCIES

Greater Vulnerability

Children are more at risk than adults to the damaging effects of radiation exposure.

Potassium Iodide Treatment

Potassium iodide treatment is only necessary in the event of exposure to radioactive iodide, which is only released from nuclear fuel (e.g., from a nuclear bomb or reactor explosions). The probability that this would be the fuel used in a dirty bomb is exceedingly small.

Children 18 and under are at the greatest risk of developing thyroid cancer after exposure to radioactive iodine. Children over 1 month of age should ideally be given potassium iodide before radioactive iodine exposure or *as soon as possible* afterward. The recommended dose of potassium iodide for children 3–18 years old is 65 mg; for children 1 month to 3 years, 32 mg; and for infants less than 1 month, 16 mg. It protects for 24 hours.

ADDITIONAL RESOURCES

American Academy of Pediatrics
    www.aap.org/terrorism and *www.aap.org/family/frk/frkit.htm*
American Red Cross: Disaster preparedness materials for children
    www.redcross.org Phone: 202-639-3520
    www.redcross.org/services/disaster/keepsafe/chemical.html#after
    www.redcross.org/services/disaster/beprepared/forchildren.html
    American Red Cross National Headquarters
    431 18th Street, NW; Washington, DC 20006
    1.   "Disaster Preparedness Coloring Book" (ARC 2200, English, or
    ARC 2200S, Spanish) Children & Disasters, ages 3–10
    2.   "Adventures of the Disaster Dudes" (ARC 5024) video and
    presenter's guide for use by an adult with children in grades 4–6
    To get copies of American Red Cross community disaster education
    materials, contact your local Red Cross chapter.
Children's Healthcare of Atlanta—Talking to Your Child About Terrorism
    (age-specific): *www.choa.org/wellchild/disaster.shtml*
Emergency Medical Service for Children—Children and post-traumatic
    stress syndrome: *www.ems-c.org/downloads/pdf/ptstress.pdf*
National Institutes of Mental Health: Helping Children and Adolescents
    Cope with Violence and Disasters
    www.nimh.nih.gov/publicat/violence.cfm
U.S. Department of Health and Human Services—Disaster Mental
    Health: *www.mentalhealth.org/cmhs/EmergencyServices/after.asp*

ANIMAL CARE

Just as you prepare yourself and your family for the event of a biological, chemical, or nuclear emergency, preparing for pet needs in advance will help protect them and enable you to act fast if you are asked to evacuate in hazardous circumstances. Many of the recommendations collected here are based on publications by the Humane Society of the United States in cooperation with the American Red Cross and by the American Veterinary Medical Association.

EMERGENCY RESPONSE

- Pets, like people, should not go outside during radiological, chemical, or most biological emergencies—especially in the event of a radiation emergency, since they could track radioactive materials from fallout back inside.

- If pets may have been contaminated, unless contamination is ongoing, thoroughly wash them with soap and water outside before bringing them inside.

EVACUATION

If you are being told to evacuate, your pets will be safest evacuating also. Even if emergency responders tell you that you will be back soon, there is no guarantee of this. However, most emergency shelters—such as those of the Red Cross—*cannot* accept animals due to state health and safety regulations. They will accept only animals that service those with disabilities. Therefore, you should explore other emergency pet options in advance:

- Find local motels and hotels in your area that will accept pets; if they do not, ask if their policy would be waived in the event of an emergency. Keep a list of these locations.

- Ask friends and relatives in the area if they would be willing to house them during an emergency.

- Prepare a list of boarding facilities and veterinarians who could shelter animals in an emergency; include 24-hour phone numbers.

- Ask local animal shelters if they provide emergency housing for animals; use as a last resort, as they could be overwhelmed in a disaster.

- Ask whether a trusted neighbor would be willing to take care of your pet should you be away from home when an evacuation order came.

Place stickers on your front and back doors and barn doors that indicate you have animals on your property, to notify neighbors and emergency personnel in case you are not at home during an evacuation.

EVACUATION KIT

Store evacuation supplies for your pet in a portable container such as a duffle bag or backpack. These should include:

- Information for nearby animal shelters
- Food and water
- Food and water bowls; can opener if needed
- Identification collar and rabies tag
- Carrier or cage
- Leash
- Medications
- Veterinary records (necessary if your pet has to go to a pet shelter)
- Information on any particular feeding schedule, medications, or behavior problems in case you need to board your pet
- Photos of your pet in case it gets lost
- Pet bed and toys, if easily transportable

SHELTERING-IN-PLACE FOR PETS

Supplies for pets to include with your home shelter-in-place supplies:

- Keep at least a 3-day food and water supply on hand for pets (ideally, keep a 2-week supply)
- Food and water bowls; can opener if needed
- Prepare a place for them to relieve themselves; garbage bags with kitty litter or newspapers could be used
- Carrier or cage
- Medications
- Pet bed and toys

MEDICAL TREATMENT

The Doctors Foster & Smith company is one online business that sells a full line of pet products, including medications. Antibiotics are available online with a prescription from a veterinarian:

Doctors Foster & Smith
www.drsfostersmith.com
Phone: 800-381-7179
P.O. Box 100
Rhinelander, WI 54501-0100

Bird medications (prescription and nonprescription):
Back Street Birds
www.backstreetbirds.com
Phone: 602-547-0946
7944 East Beck Lane, Suite 200
Scottsdale, AZ 85260

First Aid for Pets

Basic first-aid supplies should include: gauze pads, gauze roll, bandages, a roll of cloth, thermometer, tweezers, hydrogen peroxide, antibiotic ointment, Q-tips, instant cold pack, rags and rubber tubing for a tourniquet, and a first-aid manual.

Handling an Injured Animal

Any animal injured or in pain can bite or scratch you. Even the friendliest of pets must be handled with care for the safety of all involved. If you are accidentally bitten or scratched, seek medical attention. Both dog and cat bites can become infected quickly!

CARE FOR PETS OTHER THAN CATS AND DOGS

BIRDS: Birds should be transported in a secure travel cage or carrier. In cold weather, wrap a blanket over the carrier and warm up the car before placing birds inside. During warm weather, carry a plant mister to mist the birds' feathers periodically. Do not put water inside the carrier during transport. Provide a few slices of fresh fruits and vegetables with a high water content. Have a photo and leg bands for identification. If the carrier does not have a perch, line it with paper towels and change them frequently. Try to keep the carrier in a quiet area and do not let the birds out.

REPTILES: Snakes can be transported in a pillowcase but they must be transferred to more secure housing when they reach the evacuation site. If your snakes require frequent feedings, carry food with you. Take a water bowl large enough for soaking as well as a heating pad. When transporting house lizards, follow the same directions as for birds.

POCKET PETS: Small mammals (hamsters, gerbils, etc.) should be transported in secure carriers suitable for maintaining them while sheltered. Take bedding materials, food bowls, and water bottles.

ADDITIONAL RESOURCES

The American Red Cross
   www.redcross.org/services/disaster/beprepared/animalsafety.html
The American Veterinary Medical Association
   www.avma.org/vmat/disasterbrochure.asp
Animal Disaster Preparedness
   cyberpet.com/cyberdog/articles/general/artad1d.htm
Animal Management in Disasters
   www.animaldisasters.com
The Humane Society of the United States
   www.hsus.org
   2100 L Street NW
   Washington, D.C. 20037
Pet-Helpers Emergency Disaster Care
   www.pet-helpers.com
PetsWelcome: Pet-friendly lodging
   www.petswelcome.com
United Animal Nations
   www.uan.org

PREPAREDNESS AND RESPONSE SUPPLIES

An evacuation kit is a collection of portable materials you can take with you should you suddenly have to evacuate your home. Shelter-in-place materials are basic supplies that should be readily available in the event of a worst-case scenario where you are avoiding contaminants in the air and/or are required to be self-sufficient for several days. This chapter will cover these as well as home supplies and home medical treatments to prepare yourself for the biological, chemical, nuclear, and radiological emergencies discussed in this book.

TIPS FOR BOTH EVACUATION KITS AND SHELTER-IN-PLACE SUPPLIES

- Store supplies in a place easy to get to that the whole family is aware of.
- Keep items in sealed, plastic bags.
- Change most food and water supplies every 6 months.
- Canned food and unopened bottled water can be replaced once a year.
- Replace battery stores every 6 months.
- Replace stored prescription medicine as needed.

EVACUATION KIT

Evacuation-kit supplies can also serve as shelter-in-place supplies; however, evacuation supplies should be kept together in a portable container, such as a covered plastic trash bin, a camping backpack, or a duffel bag. The American Red Cross, in conjunction with the Federal Emergency Management Agency (FEMA), recommends the following items be included in an evacuation kit:

Personal Items and Supplies
Emergency preparedness manual
3-day supply of food and water
Bedding
Extra clothing (full-body coverage)
Sturdy boots or shoes
First-aid kit and manual
Essential items for people with special needs (e.g., infants, elderly, disabled)

Essential medications you are currently taking (e.g., insulin, heart medication)

Hygiene supplies

Household liquid bleach to treat drinking water

Mess kits or paper plates, cups, and plastic utensils

Manual can opener

Utility knife

Toilet paper, towelettes

Sealable plastic bags

Soap, liquid detergent

Cash or traveler's checks, change, and credit cards

Important family documents in a waterproof container

Tools

Battery-powered radio and extra batteries, or hand-crank radio

Flashlight and extra batteries

Shovel and other useful tools (e.g., screwdrivers, pliers)

Maps (regional for evacuation and local for finding public evacuation shelters)

Shovel

Tire repair kit and pump

Booster cables

Flares

Short rubber hose for siphoning

MINI-EVACUATION KIT FOR CAR

Bottled water and nonperishable, high-energy foods

Blanket or sleeping bag

Extra clothes and sturdy shoes or boots

First-aid kit and manual

Essential medications you are currently taking (e.g., insulin, heart medication)

Battery-powered radio and extra batteries, or hand-crank radio

Flashlight and extra batteries

Maps

Shovel

Tire-repair kit and pump

Booster cables

Flares

SHELTER-IN-PLACE SUPPLIES

There are seven basics that the American Red Cross and FEMA recommend you should stock for your home: water, food, sanitation provisions, first-aid supplies, clothing and bedding, tools and emergency supplies, and essential personal items. While the amount of supplies necessary to stock depends upon the event (it could be a few hours to a couple of weeks), we would recommend having enough supplies for at least 3 days, and ideally for 2 weeks or more.

Water

- Keep a **2-week supply of water** for each person in your household, which would be about **1 gallon per person per day** (2 quarts for drinking, 2 quarts for food preparation and sanitation).
- Children, nursing mothers, and the elderly will require more water than others. Hot environments and physical activity could as much as double the amount required.
- Storing unopened bottled water is recommended to ensure sanitary water. Replace once a year.
- Replace home-bottled water at least every 6 months.
- If water is not pure, you can treat it with one of the following methods:
  1. Boil for 3–5 minutes.
  2. Disinfect with 16 drops of household liquid bleach per gallon water, let stand for 15–30 minutes.
- Note that for some emergencies, water supplies may not be contaminated immediately but may become contaminated later; for this reason, you may want to fill up your bathtubs with water in case you'll need it.

Food

- Store enough nonperishable, high-energy foods to last for **2 weeks** per household member.
- Select foods that require no refrigeration, no preparation or cooking, and little or no water.
- If you must have heated food, include Sterno (canned heat cooking fuel).
- Don't stock salty foods, as they will make you thirsty.
- Replace expired food. Even canned goods should be replaced after 1 year.
- The following goods can be stored indefinitely: wheat, vegetable oils, dried corn, baking powder, soybeans, salt, noncarbonated soft drinks, white rice, bouillon products, dry pasta, powdered milk (in nitrogen-packed cans), and instant coffee, tea, and cocoa.
- You may want to include the following:
  Ready-to-eat canned meats, fruits, and vegetables
  Canned juices and prepackaged beverages
  Staples (salt, sugar, pepper, spices, etc.)

High-energy foods such as compressed protein bars, granola bars, raisins and other dried foods, trail mix, and peanut butter
Comfort foods
Vitamins

Sanitation
Toilet paper
Paper towels, moist towelettes
Soap, liquid detergent
Personal hygiene items (including feminine hygiene supplies)
Plastic garbage bags and ties (for personal sanitation use)
Plastic bucket with tight lid
Disinfectant

First-Aid Kit and Manual
First-aid kits should include sterile adhesive bandages in assorted sizes, assorted sizes of safety pins, cleansing soap, latex gloves, sunscreen, sterile gauze pads, triangular bandages, sterile roller bandages, scissors, tweezers, a needle, moistened towelettes, antiseptic, thermometer, tongue blades, petroleum jelly or other lubricant

Tools
Battery-powered radio and extra batteries, or hand-crank radio
Flashlight and extra batteries
Manual can opener
Utility knife
Fire extinguisher (5 lb., A–B–C type)
Shutoff wrench to turn off household gas or water
Pliers, screwdrivers, hammer, nails, and other useful tools
Matches in a waterproof container
Plastic storage containers
Aluminum foil
Medicine dropper
Needle and thread
Whistle
Compass
You may want to include a portable heater if in a cold climate
You may want to include a portable generator with gasoline supply; note that you must vent the exhaust outside to prevent carbon monoxide poisoning

Other Essentials

Emergency preparedness manual

Essential items for people with special needs (e.g., infants, elderly, disabled)

Essential medications you are currently taking (e.g., insulin, heart medication)

Extra eyeglasses or contact lenses and cleaning supplies

Bedding

Clothing for warm, cold, and rainy weather; include at least one outfit of full-body coverage for each member of the household

Towels

Household liquid bleach to treat drinking water

Mess kits or paper plates, cups, and plastic utensils (disposable to conserve water)

Sealable plastic bags

Signal flare

Telephone or cell phone

Entertainment

Baby Needs

Formula

Baby food

Diapers

Medicines

Bottles

Powdered milk

Pets

See Chapter 32, *Animal Care*

HOME SUPPLIES FOR BIOLOGICAL, CHEMICAL, AND NUCLEAR EMERGENCIES

Household liquid chlorine bleach (sodium hypochlorite, 5%) without other ingredients

Germicide soap

Disinfectant for furniture and other surfaces

Duct tape

Garbage bags or plastic sheeting (for sealing shelter)

Goggles (such as swim goggles) for eye protection for each household member

HEPA (high-efficiency particle arresting) filters for ventilation systems: HEPA filters were developed by the U.S. government to protect scientists from radioactive airborne particles. They remove 99.97%

of particles 0.3 microns and smaller, which includes dust, mold spores, dust mites, pet dander, allergens, and many biological agents such as anthrax spores. Note that HEPA filters do not purify the air of most chemical agents.

HEPA filters for vacuum cleaners

Insect repellent

Latex gloves

Respiratory Masks

– All masks for respiratory protection should be approved by the National Institute for Occupational Safety and Health (NIOSH) and will say so on their boxes.

– Note that, in general, facial hair greatly reduces the fit and thus the effectiveness of respiratory masks.

– Disposable surgical respiratory masks (nonfiltered fiber masks) are only effective for protecting against relatively large particles, such as dust.

– N95 disposable respiratory masks cost about $1 each (recommended).

– N100 disposable respiratory masks are 5% more effective than N95s and cost about $5 each.

– N100 elastomeric masks are even better than N95 and N- or P100 masks to protect against biological agents; they can be purchased at hardware stores for about $20 and have filters that cost about $5 each.

– The only types of respiratory masks that are effective for chemical agents are gas masks. Military-type gas masks that protect against chemicals are not rated by NIOSH for use because they physically restrict breathing and could harm the untrained user. Professional hazardous-materials personnel usually wear highly sophisticated "supplied-air respirators," which involve a tank that supplies clean air.

OVER-THE-COUNTER MEDICINES AND TREATMENTS FOR BIOLOGICAL, CHEMICAL, AND NUCLEAR EMERGENCIES

Activated charcoal

Antacid for stomach upset

Antidiarrhea medication

Antihistamines

Antinausea medication

Aspirin and nonaspirin pain relievers (e.g., acetaminophen)

Betadine (povodine iodine) as a topical antiseptic for skin and for blister agent treatment

Laxative

Oral rehydration solutions (e.g., Pedialyte, Gatorade)

Potassium iodide

Saline wash for eyes

Syrup of ipecac (to induce vomiting if instructed to do so by your doctor)

SELF-PRESCRIBING ANTIBIOTICS

Do *not* begin drug treatment until you have been instructed to do so by an authorized medical professional. It is extremely important to keep in mind the following precautions:

- Unnecessary and frequent use of antibiotics could kill the weakest bacteria and leave the strongest to keep reproducing and infecting others. In this way, we could build antibiotic-resistant bacteria, or bacteria that cannot be killed by common (or possibly any) antibiotics.
- Sophisticated laboratories could develop bacteria that are resistant to certain antibiotics that would normally kill them, hence you need specific medical direction on a case-by-case basis.
- Allergic reactions to antibiotics are not uncommon and can even be life-threatening.
- Many antibiotics have special precautions for children, pregnant women, and people with certain medical conditions.
- Antibiotics may cross-react with other medications you are taking.

For these reasons, we do not recommend that you self-administer antibiotics; consult your physician beforehand.

In the biological-weapons chapters, antibiotics are listed as the primary treatment for all of the bacterial diseases. It is important to note that often the first-choice treatment in the event of an outbreak for patients with established infection and significant symptoms is for antibiotics to be given directly into a vein (intravenously, IV) or into the muscle (intramuscularly, IM)—the sort of drug therapy dispersed from a hospital. If there is a bioterrorist attack of great magnitude, the healthcare system may be too overwhelmed to administer drugs by IV or IM. In this case, oral antibiotics (by mouth) would be recommended. In cases of an outbreak where protective antibiotic dosages are given to a population (called prophylaxis), the antibiotics would also be oral dosages.

ONLINE MEDICATIONS: FRAUD ALERT

In conjunction with the Centers for Disease Control and Prevention (CDC) and the Food and Drug Administration (FDA), the Federal Trade Commission (FTC) warns consumers against fraudsters that offer prescription medications online, preying on consumers' fears and vulnerabilities. They offer the following advice:

- **Talk to your healthcare professional before you use any medications.** Confirming an infection requires a doctor's examination and diagnosis.
- **Know that some websites may sell ineffective drugs.** Some sites may claim to sell FDA-approved drugs, like ciprofloxacin ("cipro"), made to meet U.S. standards. In fact, the drugs could be counterfeit or even adulterated with dangerous contaminants.
- **Know whom you are buying from.** Online, anyone can pretend to be anyone. To ensure that the site is reputable and licensed to sell drugs in the United States, the FDA recommends that you check with the National Association of Boards of Pharmacy at *www.nabp.net*, or at phone number 847-698-6227, to determine whether a website is a licensed pharmacy in good standing.
- **In addition, the FTC and FDA caution:**
  - Don't buy prescription drugs from sites that offer to prescribe them without a physical exam, sell drugs without a prescription, or sell drugs unapproved by the FDA.
  - Don't do business with websites that don't give you access to pharmacists to answer questions.
  - Avoid sites that don't provide their name, physical business address, and phone number.
  - Don't purchase from foreign websites. It is generally illegal to import drugs that are sold by these sites; the risks are greater, and there is very little the U.S. government can do if you are taken advantage of.
  - If you buy drugs online, pay by credit or charge card.

For more information from the federal government about treatments for anthrax and other diseases, visit *www.consumer.gov*. For more information from the FDA, call toll-free 1-800-INFO-FDA or visit *www.fda.gov*. Information on bioterrorism and public-health preparedness from the CDC is available at *www.bt.cdc.gov* and also by telephone at 1-800-311-3435. To file a complaint or to get free information on consumer issues, call the FTC toll-free at 1-877-FTC-HELP, or use the complaint form at *www.ftc.gov*.

Introduction to Mass Transportation

Though in the United States we had been mostly spared from attacks upon our transportation system until September 11, 2001, terrorists abroad have used weapons to kill and injure civilians on mass transportation for decades. Post–September 11, U.S. authorities have issued several general warnings of possible terrorist attacks on parts of the transportation system across the United States, including airplanes, trains and railroads, subways, ships, and bridges.

Many new transportation security measures have been put into place and billions of government dollars allotted for this purpose since September 11. One of the most significant changes is the passage of the Aviation and Transportation Security Act, which President George W. Bush signed into law on November 19, 2001, creating the Transportation Security Administration (TSA) within the Department of Transportation. Though the emphasis is currently on upgrading aviation security, the TSA will be dedicated to the prevention of attacks by criminals or terrorists against any form of commercial transportation or infrastructure, including America's highways, waterways, seaports, railways, public transit, and pipelines. The TSA will work with all of the U.S. government agencies to gather and share intelligence information. They plan to design and operate a system of integrated, overlapping, national security systems—some of which will be visible to the public, and others of which will not.

GENERAL PRECAUTIONS

Suspicious Package

If you discover an abandoned or unattended bag, box, backpack, or any other type of container left in or near a public or private space, do not touch, open, or move it, and keep your distance! The majority of unattended packages are harmless—however, if you find a suspicious package, contact your local police or 911 immediately. Characteristics of suspicious packages may include:

- Unusual batteries or protruding wires or aluminum foil
- Tanks, bottles, or bags indicating the presence of a chemical
- A message attached to the article
- Suspicious clouds, mists, gases, vapors, or odors
- The appearance of something seeping from the article
- The observation of someone abandoning the article and leaving quickly
- Finding the article in an out-of-the way place
- A ticking sound

If at work, notify a supervisor, a security officer, the facility manager, or police (911). Do not report a suspicious package by radio or cellular phone unless you are more than 300 feet from the incident location. When reporting, be prepared to provide detailed information about what activity is taking place, where it is taking place, and the individuals who are involved.

Emergency Response on Mass Transportation

Announcements during emergencies: All transportation systems provide emergency and disaster training for their personnel in coordination with local emergency management agencies. No matter what the situation, always listen for announcements and follow instructions from transportation personnel and/or emergency service personnel. Following instructions and staying calm and orderly can prevent further injuries and save lives.

Below are general emergency steps to follow for all mass-transportation incidents that involve an aerosol release of unknown substance or an explosion:

- *Stay calm.*
- Follow instructions from the operator, crew members, or emergency personnel.
- Cover your mouth and nose with fabric, wet if possible. Remember that explosive devices may be designed to disseminate biological, chemical, or radioactive agents.
- For possible biological incidents, wear a respiratory mask if you have one.
- Breathe in as little as possible until you are out of the area; take shallow breaths.
- Cover exposed skin.
- If your eyes are burning, try to keep them closed unless it inhibits your escape.
- Leave the area, going *against the wind* and *uphill*.
- If there is no one to assist you, remove outer clothing and wash off with plenty of water, then wait for emergency personnel.
- Decontamination and medical evaluation may be required once you are away from the hazardous area.

For detailed response recommendations, see the following
EMERGENCY RESPONSE **sections:**

Airborne spray causing no obvious symptoms	Chapter 16, *Unidentified Biological Agent*
Chemical attack / people suddenly falling ill	Chapter 24, *Unidentified Chemical Agent*
Bomb or explosion	Chapter 29, *Event with Unknown Radioactivity*

AIRPLANES

ASSESSMENT OF RISK

Because of greatly increased airline security measures, the chances of an airplane hijacking or bomb detonation are much reduced since September 11; however, the system is not perfect. Experts say there are simply too many airports and commercial flights in the United States to ensure that determined terrorists, particularly those willing to commit suicide, will not find a way to use an aircraft in a future attack. There is a long list of terrorist bombings aboard aircraft around the world: in the last 30 years, more than 33 countries and 40 airlines were victims of terrorism of this sort. Nevertheless, it is worth remembering that, statistically, air travel remains far safer than any other form of transportation.

CURRENT SECURITY MEASURES IN PLACE

Here are some of the steps that the new Aviation and Transportation Security Act put into effect to help secure our airports and planes:

- It created the Transportation Security Administration (TSA), a new federal agency within the Department of Transportation, most of whose efforts and resources so far have been devoted to overseeing airport and airline security.
- It required that all U.S. airport security be handled by federal employees, including those monitoring baggage and passengers, by November 18, 2002 (which it has done).
- It mandated that by December 31, 2002, all airports be equipped with explosive-detection systems that will screen all checked bags for bombs and explosives. (Though only two companies are certified to make these systems and each one costs about $1 million, the deadline was almost met. Congress authorized extensions to a handful of the nation's airports, which will use other congressionally approved screening methods in the interim.)
- It called for fortified cockpit doors, more plainclothes air marshals aboard planes, and mandatory training for flight crews about how to handle a hijacking.

Additional security enhancements include limiting carry-on luggage to one bag and one personal item per passenger; allowing only ticketed passengers past security checkpoints; removing luggage checked on planes if the passenger who checked it does not board; confiscating sharp implements found on a person or in carry-on luggage; and searching more passengers and their carry-on luggage at the gates.

Federal Air Marshals (originally called "sky marshals") are armed and trained in combat, marksmanship, effective use of minimal force, and terrorist strategies. They are fully qualified to respond to incidents aboard aircraft. Out of the tens of thousands of flights every day in the United States, there are thousands of Federal Air Marshals flying on them, and their numbers are increasing. Pilots are currently not authorized to carry firearms on flights, although this may change.

Computer-Assisted Passenger Prescreening System (CAPPS) is a computer program that uses a set of secret criteria to identify passengers who might be dangerous. For example, CAPPS singled out six of the September 11 hijackers—however, unfortunately, this only resulted in more thorough screening of their checked baggage. Passengers identified by CAPPS are now pulled aside and closely scrutinized, and both their carry-on and checked baggage is thoroughly searched.

The National Guard, in addition to supplementing the U.S. Armed Forces, has the role of assisting civil leaders during natural disasters, civil unrest, and state emergencies. They were called upon to protect civilian airports post-9/11, but they have been phased out since spring of 2002. The Transportation Security Administration federal screeners and supervisors have now taken their place. The National Guard remains active in emergency- and disaster-response training in the event that they are needed again.

The Animal and Plant Health Inspection Service (APHIS) (of the U.S. Department of Agriculture) has a presence at airports to monitor biological and animal transportation.

EMERGENCY RESOURCES FOR PASSENGERS

Safety features that may be present:
- Oxygen masks that drop from overhead
- White lights on the floor or aisle seats that light the aisle in the event of an emergency; red lights indicate an exit
- Emergency doors in the passenger cabin that can be manually removed by an able-bodied person
- Inflatable slides at the base of most emergency exits
- Most seat bottoms are designed to serve as flotation devices
- Inflatable life jackets (may be under the seat or between seats)
- Inflatable life rafts (may be behind a panel in a ceiling compartment)

- Fire extinguishers
- Medical kits including oxygen, other medical supplies, and possibly an automatic external defibrillator

AIRBORNE SPRAY CAUSING NO OBVIOUS SYMPTOMS

- An airborne spray causing no obvious symptoms may be a biological agent. It may also be a hoax or scare tactic.
- If you use an oxygen mask dropped from the ceiling, continuously press it tightly over your mouth and nose, as it will not fit securely otherwise. Seal the cup with a wet cloth if possible.
- Bear in mind that most infectious agents do not have immediate lethal effects and are treatable.

CHEMICAL ATTACK / PEOPLE SUDDENLY FALLING ILL

- Move as far from the release site as possible.
- If you use an oxygen mask dropped from the ceiling, continuously press it tightly over your mouth and nose, as it will not fit securely otherwise. Seal the cup with a wet cloth if possible.
- Remove outer clothing and rinse skin with water or liquid if a chemical agent is suspected.
- If your eyes are burning, keep them closed.

BOMB OR EXPLOSION

- Of the airplane bombings of the last 30 years (40 airlines in 33 countries), on average 56% of the aircraft survived the in-flight bombing (73% for wide-bodied aircraft and 48% for narrow-bodied).
- A breach in the cabin will necessitate breathing from an oxygen mask until pilots bring the plane down to 10,000 feet or lower.

SHOOTING

If bullets punctured a pressurized cabin, the holes would be so small that dangerous decompression would be unlikely. Computers controlling the air pressure would compensate for the change in pressure. Even if bullets hit a crucial piece of equipment, airplanes are equipped with much redundancy so that if one aspect fails, something either compensates or a second unit exists altogether, especially for the most vital functions. An opening the size of a cabin window or larger, however, could cause problems but probably would not be catastrophic to the aircraft (see "Decompression" in the *OTHER EMERGENCIES* section below).

HIJACKING

- The U.S. Department of State's Bureau of Consular Affairs offers the following advice specifically for hostage situations:
  - The most dangerous phases of a hijacking or hostage situation are usually the beginning and, if there is a rescue attempt, the end. At the outset, the terrorists typically are tense, high-strung, and may behave irrationally. It is extremely important that you remain calm and alert and manage your own behavior.
  - Avoid resistance and sudden or threatening movements. Do not struggle or try to escape unless you are certain of being successful.
  - Make a concerted effort to relax.
  - Try to remain inconspicuous. Avoid direct eye contact and the appearance of watching your captors' actions.
  - Put yourself in a mode of passive cooperation. Talk normally. Do not complain. Avoid belligerence; comply with all orders and instructions.
  - If questioned, keep your answers short. Don't volunteer information or make unnecessary overtures.
  - Don't try to be a hero, endangering yourself and others.
  - Think positively. Avoid a sense of despair. Rely on your inner resources. Remember that most often you are a valuable commodity to your captors. For most hostage takers, keeping you alive and well is important.
- In an event that appears similar to a 9/11 hijacking in which everyone will perish unless action is taken, Ken Cubbin, author of *Survival Tactics for Airline Passengers*, suggests the following:
  - Be alert to others in the cabin. Observe suspicious or nervous behavior, including a passenger who wants to talk to the pilot.
  - Check your seat neighbors for possible allies.
  - If suspicious behavior becomes an obvious, full-blown threat, shout, "Help! Help! Help!" as loud as you can.
  - Quickly tell the cabin passengers to form a group.
  - Do not obey terrorist orders to herd to the back of the plane.
  - Do not be intimidated by bomb threats or weapons. You're not alone.
  - Shout for everyone to throw objects at the assailants' heads. Use anything you can, such as laptops, full soda cans, bags, heavy shoes, and trays. Keep up a steady barrage.
  - Rapidly gang-rush the assailants as a group. Crush them to the floor and restrain them.

  In addition:
  - You can use a tightly rolled magazine as a weapon.
  - You can use seat cushions as a shield when rushing assailants.
  - Wrap clothing around your arms to protect yourself from assailants slashing.

OTHER EMERGENCIES

- **Decompression:** Above around 8,000 feet, oxygen in the air begins to thin out, so a plane draws this air in and compresses it inside the cabin to create comfortable breathing air. Thus, a "decompressed" cabin occurs if the fuselage is breached, as the highly pressurized air inside the cabin rushes outside. If this happens, oxygen masks will automatically drop from overhead. If the decompression is serious, pilots will make an emergency drop to 10,000 feet, a descent that could be bumpy. Fog may appear in the cabin as the outside air replaces the compressed air and the temperature drops. If the opening is large, decompression may be violent and carry objects and people out with the rush of air. For example, a Boeing-747 flying near Hawaii had a cargo door and large section of the fuselage blow out, taking nine passengers with it. Another decompression occurred when one-third of the roof of a Boeing-737 ripped off in flight; a passenger who had been walking through the cabin at the time was lost. Both planes were able to land safely.

- **Water Landings:** Airplanes are designed to float and float high enough such that emergency exits remain above the waterline.

- **Engine Failure:** Most commercial airliners are equipped with two fully functioning engines. For every thousand feet of altitude, a large aircraft can glide for one mile or more. Pilots can maneuver the flight controls and land without power if they can make it to a suitable landing area (as happened in a trans-Atlantic flight in 2001).

EVACUATION

- Airplanes are designed for easy evacuation. To certify a new airplane of 44 seats or more, the Federal Aviation Administration (FAA) requires that all passengers and crew be able to exit within 90 seconds, even with half the exits blocked.
- If there is smoke, stay low to the ground and cover your mouth with fabric, such as a pillowcase or headrest, and wet it if you can.
- Stay calm, and follow the instructions of the crew members.
- Do not take carry-on baggage with you—it will slow you and everybody else down.
- Remember: "White lights lead to red lights." Follow white lights on the floor or side of the aisle seats to red lights, which indicate an exit.
- Just as pre-flight reminders instruct, remember that the closest exit may be behind you.
- Climb over seats if the aisle is blocked.
- Get as far away from the plane as you can when you are out. Even if the plane appears fine, there may be fuel leaks and open electrical circuitry if the plane has been damaged.

BUSES

ASSESSMENT OF RISK

Since September 11, U.S. authorities have issued several general warnings of possible terrorist attacks on parts of the ground transportation system. Unlike airplanes, where passengers and luggage are screened beforehand at security checkpoints, buses are designed to be easily accessible and are therefore harder to protect. Countless terrorists in other countries have targeted buses in the past, both by leaving packages containing an improvised explosive device (IED)/bomb in them or in suicide missions with bombs strapped to their bodies.

CURRENT SECURITY MEASURES IN PLACE

Greyhound Lines, America's largest provider of bus transportation between cities, has expanded pre- and post-trip checks of vehicles and is using more security guards and cameras, as well as metal-detecting wands to inspect passengers at some locations.

Metro Buses

- Some buses, such as Metrobuses in Washington, D.C., and in New York City, have silent alarms that the bus operator can activate in an emergency situation with a threatening passenger. The alarm goes through Central Control to the police, the destination sign on the outside of the bus changes to "EMERGENCY! CALL POLICE," and the outside running lights flash to let approaching police know which bus sent out the alarm, all unbeknownst to the disruptive passenger(s).
- Undercover and uniformed police officers travel on some bus routes (as they do in New York City).

EMERGENCY RESOURCES FOR PASSENGERS

Safety features that may be present:

Emergency windows

Emergency-exit procedures listed on windows, ceiling escape hatches, and doors

Fire extinguishers (may be located inside the front door under the passenger-side seat or beneath/behind the driver's seat)

Emergency door release

AIRBORNE SPRAY CAUSING NO OBVIOUS SYMPTOMS
- An airborne spray causing no obvious symptoms may be a biological agent. It may also be a hoax or scare tactic.
- Get off the bus immediately.
- If you're not able to get off, open as many windows as possible.

CHEMICAL ATTACK / PEOPLE SUDDENLY FALLING ILL
- Get off the bus immediately.
- If you're not able to get off, move away from the dispersal site and open as many windows as possible.
- If there is no one to assist you, remove outer clothing and find a place to wash off right away, then seek help from emergency personnel.

BOMB OR EXPLOSION
- Get off the bus as soon as it stops and get far away from it. There is always the possibility of a secondary explosion.
- If exiting through smoke, keep close to the ground and cover your mouth with fabric (wet if possible).
- Once away from the immediate area, wait for emergency personnel to assist you.

HIJACKING
- Some buses have silent/panic alarms that the bus operator can activate in an emergency situation with a threatening passenger. Undetectable to bus passengers, the alarm may secretly alert police or the bus command center by radio, change the destination sign on the outside of the bus to "EMERGENCY! CALL POLICE," and/or flash outside running lights to identify the bus to authorities.
- In an extreme situation, such as an event similar to 9/11 in which everyone will perish unless action is taken, lives may be saved by bus passengers coming together to overthrow the hijackers. (See the hijacking section in Chapter 34, *Airplanes*, for more detailed recommendations.)

EVACUATION
- Stay calm, and follow the instructions of the bus operator.
- Climb over seats if the aisle is blocked.
- Most buses can be exited via emergency windows and ceiling escape hatches if need be. Emergency windows are designed in several ways, but most either push out or slide across after an emergency lever is released. Breaking today's bus windows is neither possible nor practical.

CRUISE SHIPS

ASSESSMENT OF RISK

Modern-day cruise ships can carry 5,000 passengers and crew members. Hence, they may be a target for terrorists since a successful attack on one of these ships could result in a catastrophic number of casualties, in addition to threatening the economic viability of the industry. However, following the events of September 11, 2001, all cruise ship lines, cruise vessels, and cruise terminals have been in a heightened state of alert (see below).

CURRENT SECURITY MEASURES IN PLACE

The United States Coast Guard, which oversees cruise vessels and ports in U.S. territories, has initiated a directive for all cruise vessel operations to be at the highest security level since 9/11. These additional measures of security include:

- Screening of all baggage and cargo, including by x-ray, prior to boarding
- Screening of all passengers and carry-on items prior to boarding
- Confirmation of each passenger against the official passenger list before boarding
- Confirmation of all baggage against the official passenger list before it is boarded
- Increased number of guards and/or intrusion-detection systems (IDS) at all terminals and vessel-restricted areas
- The enforcing of a 300-foot separation zone around all cruise vessels while in port and en route into and out of port
- The escorting of all cruise vessels into and out of port

Other measures may include:

- Private security officers on board
- Guest manifest checked against FBI and Immigration Naturalization Services (INS) computers and matched for suspects
- Background checks for crew
- Inspections for explosives
- Guests pass through metal detectors at every port of call
- X-ray of all port-of-call items brought on the vessel
- Divers sent to inspect the hull at every port

EMERGENCY RESOURCES FOR PASSENGERS

Life rafts

Life jackets

Fire hoses and extinguishers

In addition to first aid, large ships should have an infirmary and medical staff, lifesaving equipment, and prescription drugs

BIOLOGICAL TERRORISM

Cruise ships are a perfect breeding ground for contagious diseases. Isolating large groups of people and putting them together in the closed environment of a ship at sea greatly increases the chances for person-to-person spread of diseases, especially certain respiratory and gastrointestinal illnesses. It is for these reasons that it is not all that uncommon for natural outbreaks of diseases to occur on these vessels. It is also for these reasons that a deliberate attack could have far-reaching consequences. The Centers for Disease Control monitors illness outbreaks on cruise ships. See Chapter 16, *Unidentified Biological Agent*, for specific precautions you can take.

AIRBORNE SPRAY CAUSING NO OBVIOUS SYMPTOMS

- An airborne spray causing no obvious symptoms may be a biological agent. It may also be a hoax or scare tactic.
- Unless instructed otherwise, on deck in the open air is probably the safest place to go. Stay upwind of the release area.

CHEMICAL ATTACK / PEOPLE SUDDENLY FALLING ILL

- Try not to breathe in until you are out of the area where people are falling ill.
- Move as far from an airborne spray release site as you can. Do not go through a chemical spray or vapors if at all possible, even quickly.
- Unless instructed otherwise, on deck in the open air is probably the safest place to go. Move upwind of the release area.
- If there is no one to assist you in decontamination, remove outer clothing and find a place to wash off right away, then seek help from crew members.

BOMB OR EXPLOSION

- Move as far away from the explosion site as you can. Do not walk through the site if possible.
- Be extremely vigilant about your surroundings: terrorists may have additional bombs ready to detonate.

- If exiting through smoke, keep close to the ground and cover your mouth with fabric (wet if possible).
- A large enough breach in the hull could sink even a giant cruise ship. Listen for evacuation instructions.

SHOOTING
- The Department of State's Bureau of Consular Affairs recommends the following if you are ever in a situation where somebody starts shooting:
  - Drop to the floor or get down as low as possible.
  - Don't move until you are sure the danger has passed.
  - Do not attempt to help rescuers, and do not pick up a weapon.
  - If possible, shield yourself behind or under a solid object.
  - If you must move, crawl on your stomach.

HIJACKING

Hijacking a cruise ship is not unprecedented: in 1985 four heavily armed Palestinian terrorists commandeered the Italian cruise ship *Achille Lauro* in the Mediterranean Sea for two days, killing an American tourist.

The State Department offers the following advice specifically for hostage situations:
  - The most dangerous phases of a hijacking or hostage situation are usually the beginning and, if there is a rescue attempt, the end. At the outset, the terrorists typically are tense, high-strung, and may behave irrationally. It is extremely important that you remain calm and alert and manage your own behavior.
  - Avoid resistance and sudden or threatening movements. Do not struggle or try to escape unless you are certain of being successful.
  - Make a concerted effort to relax. Prepare yourself mentally, physically, and emotionally for the possibility of a long ordeal.
  - Try to remain inconspicuous. Avoid direct eye contact and the appearance of watching your captors' actions.
  - Put yourself in a mode of passive cooperation. Talk normally. Do not complain. Avoid belligerence, and comply with all orders and instructions.
  - If questioned, keep your answers short. Don't volunteer information or make unnecessary overtures.
  - Don't try to be a hero, endangering yourself and others.
  - If you are involved in a lengthier, drawn-out situation, try to establish a rapport with your captors, avoiding political discussions or other confrontational subjects.

- Maintain your sense of personal dignity, and gradually increase your requests for personal comforts. Make these requests in a reasonable, low-key manner.
- Establish a daily program of mental and physical activity. Don't be afraid to ask for anything you need or want, such as medicines, books, pencils, and papers.
- Eat what they give you, even if it does not look or taste appetizing.
- Think positively. Avoid a sense of despair. Rely on your inner resources. Remember that you are a valuable commodity to your captors. It is important to them to keep you alive and well.

EVACUATION

Evacuation on cruise ships is well planned and is tailored to each individual ship. Emergency-evacuation drills conducted on the ships prepare and familiarize passengers in procedures for evacuations. Read safety manuals at the beginning of the trip. Listen carefully for instructions from crew members.

SUBWAYS

ASSESSMENT OF RISK

Since September 11, U.S. authorities have issued several general warnings of possible terrorist attacks on parts of the ground transportation system, including subways. Unlike airplanes, where passengers and luggage are screened beforehand at security checkpoints, mass transit is easily accessible and therefore harder to protect. Subway systems are particularly vulnerable because of their relatively small, enclosed areas (both the cars and stations), which become crowded at predictable times during the day, such as rush hour. In addition, air currents from above ground and underground, generated by movement of trains through the tunnels, could spread germs or gases throughout a subway system—and through ventilation systems to the streets above—leading to the infection/contamination of large numbers of people. Furthermore, because symptoms of exposure to some biological agents would not appear for a couple of weeks, victims could unknowingly leave the station and infect many others.

In the 1960s the CIA and the U.S. Army conducted a test in which lightbulbs filled with microscopic particles (a harmless form of anthrax) were dropped between moving subway cars onto the New York City subway tracks to measure the possible effects of a biological attack. The study suggested that a similar type of attack using a deadly disease agent such as tularemia would have infected as many as 3 million people.

CURRENT SECURITY MEASURES IN PLACE

- Increased police presence, including undercover officers
- Increased government funding for security improvements
- The government is helping agencies assess preparedness and identify vulnerabilities; refine emergency response plans; coordinate response efforts with firefighters, police, and other emergency personnel; conduct emergency drills to keep skills and response plans up-to-date; and train transit employees to understand current security issues and respond to these emergencies
- In Washington, D.C., subway trash receptacles are being replaced with bomb-resistant cans
- In New York City, suspicious packages are now regularly investigated and x-rayed

- Chemical, biological, and radiological sensing machines are being installed (these are rare)

EMERGENCY RESOURCES FOR PASSENGERS
The following safety features may be present:
- Emergency brakes*
- Emergency door releases
- Station booth agents have phones to contact emergency medical services and the police
- Train operators (usually in the first car) and train conductors (usually in a middle car) have radios to call their rail command center for help
- Fire extinguishers, usually located in the ends of cars

* The only reason to pull an emergency brake is for a runaway train where confirmation has been made that the train operator is not capable of controlling the train. Under all other circumstances do not pull the brake, but listen to crew members' instructions.

AIRBORNE SPRAY CAUSING NO OBVIOUS SYMPTOMS
- An airborne spray causing no obvious symptoms may be a biological agent. It may also be a hoax or scare tactic.
- Move out of the car of exposure; do not walk through the spray if you can avoid it.
- Remain on the train if between stations, and open as many windows as possible.
- Get off at the next station, and follow instructions of the train crew.
- Bear in mind that most infectious agents do not have immediate lethal effects and are treatable.

CHEMICAL ATTACK / PEOPLE SUDDENLY FALLING ILL
- Move as far from an airborne spray release site as you can. Do not go through a chemical spray or vapors if at all possible.
- If you have to go through the hazardous area, hold your breath and proceed as quickly as possible. Once in the next car, remove outer clothing and, if possible, flush with copious amounts of water. (Note, the safest place to ride a subway may be a center car, since, assuming there is only one dispersal site, you will always have an escape direction.)
- Do *not* activate the train's emergency brake. Once the brake is pulled, the train will stop, thus preventing emergency personnel from reaching sick passengers.

- Do not get out of the train between stations—in most all circumstances you are safer on the train: outside, trains may be traveling on adjacent tracks, and the third rail may still be electrified.
- If you need to open the exit doors, there should be an emergency exit panel with clearly labeled instructions.
- If you cannot exit through the side doors or need to open the windows for ventilation, open the clearly marked emergency window exits. Opening an emergency window usually requires pulling a red handle at the top to remove the rubber molding that holds it in place, then pulling a second handle on the glass toward you to remove the window.
- Get off right away at the next stop and *leave the station*, going against the wind and uphill. Most chemical agents that might be used in an attack are heavier than air so would linger underground. Note that before trains are stopped and ventilation systems turned off, a chemical gas would continue to flow to adjacent underground stations.
- If there is no one to assist you, remove outer clothing and find a place to wash off right away, then seek help from emergency responders.

BOMB OR EXPLOSION

- Move as far away from the explosion site as you can. Do not walk through the site if possible.
- Be extremely vigilant of your surroundings: terrorists may have a second bomb ready to detonate.
- If exiting through smoke, keep close to the ground and cover your mouth with fabric (wet if possible).
- Do not activate the emergency brake in the event of a fire or explosion, especially in tunnels. Once the brake is pulled, the brakes have to be reset before the train can move again, thus increasing the time it takes for fire, police, and medical services to respond to the incident. Use the emergency brake only when the forward motion of the train presents an imminent danger to life and limb.
- If between stations, stay on the train if at all possible since track areas are very dangerous.
- If you need to open the exit doors, there should be an emergency exit panel with clearly labeled instructions.
- If you cannot exit through the side doors or need to open the windows for ventilation, open the clearly marked emergency window exits. Opening an emergency window usually requires pulling a red handle at the top to remove the rubber molding that holds it in place, then pulling a second handle on the glass toward you to remove the window.

EVACUATION

- Do not attempt to leave the train without help from the train crew: outside, trains may be traveling on adjacent tracks, and the third rail may still be electrified. In most circumstances, leaving the train is the most dangerous thing you can do.
- For subways with catenary cables (overhead contact power lines), the above applies if the lines are down or near the ground.
- Climb over seats if the aisle is blocked.
- If you need to open the exit doors, there should be an emergency exit panel with clearly labeled instructions.
- If you cannot exit through the side doors, open the clearly marked emergency windows. Opening an emergency window usually requires pulling a red handle at the top to remove the rubber molding that holds it in place, then pulling a second handle on the glass toward you to remove the window.
- If you have to exit the train between stations:
  - Do not touch tracks or cables.
  - Utilize catwalks to exit tunnel areas if possible.
  - You may find an emergency exit between stations; if not, continue to the next station.
  - Exit into the street, and move against the wind and uphill.

TRAINS

This chapter refers to ABOVE-GROUND TRAINS and includes long-distance passenger trains (e.g., Amtrak) as well as commuter trains.

ASSESSMENT OF RISK

Since September 11, U.S. authorities have issued several general warnings of possible terrorist attacks on parts of the ground transportation system, including trains and railroads. Unlike airplanes, where passengers and luggage are screened beforehand at security checkpoints, passenger trains are designed to be easily accessible and are therefore harder to protect. Ground-transportation systems, which often involve enclosed spaces crowded with people (i.e., train cars and terminals), could prove to be tempting targets for terrorists.

Freight trains: Warnings have been sent by Homeland Security officials to U.S. railroads mentioning potential threats to freight trains, in particular regarding threats to bridges, engines, and hazardous-materials cars. Release of hazardous materials in a heavily populated area could cause mass casualties and necessitate widespread environmental cleanup. The rail industry has stepped up security measures since 9/11. This chapter will focus on passenger trains.

CURRENT SECURITY MEASURES IN PLACE

AMTRAK's new security precautions taken post–September 11:
- Carry-on luggage is limited to two pieces
- All checked baggage must have identification tags
- Three hundred-some uniformed and undercover police officers regularly ride the trains
- Tickets bought at automated tellers are matched against FBI watch lists
- Increased government funding for security improvements

COMMUTER TRAINS may have:
- Closed-circuit video cameras monitoring stations
- Central command station with computer display showing precise location of every train and a hotline to police and fire departments
- Chemical or radiological sensing machines (very new, still rare)
- Increased police presence, including undercover officers
- Increased government funding for security improvements and drills

EMERGENCY RESOURCES FOR PASSENGERS

AMTRAK trains may have the following (often located at train car junctions):

Emergency brakes*
Emergency exit ("side") door release handles
Emergency windows
Fire extinguishers
First-aid kits
Emergency tools
Snaplights (sticks that illuminate when broken)
Emergency ladders
Emergency communication boxes for communication with train personnel to officials outside the train

COMMUTER TRAINS may have:

Emergency brakes*
Emergency intercoms ("call boxes") at either end of each car as well as on station platforms, connecting with train operators
Emergency door releases (may be in a call box or at the base of the seat closest to the door; it may say "Emergency Exit Panel")
Fire extinguishers located in the operator's cab and may be available under the last row of seats at the end of the car
Emergency call boxes along the tracks (e.g., they are every 800 feet in Washington, D.C.); may be marked by blue lights and have a button that can shut down the third rail in extreme emergencies
Station-booth agents have phones to contact emergency medical services and the police
Newer trains may have public phones with credit-card access

* The only reason to pull an emergency brake is for a runaway train where confirmation has been made that the train operator is not capable of controlling the train. Under all other circumstances do not pull the brake, but listen to crew member instructions.

AIRBORNE SPRAY CAUSING NO OBVIOUS SYMPTOMS

- An airborne spray causing no obvious symptoms may be a biological agent. It may also be a hoax or scare tactic.
- Leave the area of dispersal—do not walk through the spray if you can avoid it—and go to the farthest car that you can reach. Try not to breathe until you are out of the vicinity.
- If you're unable to leave the train car, open windows.
- Wait for instructions from the train crew or emergency personnel.

– Do *not* activate the train's emergency brake, especially in a tunnel. Once the brake is pulled, the brakes have to be reset before the train can move again, thus increasing the time it takes for fire, police, and medical services to respond to the incident.

– For COMMUTER TRAINS, get off at the next station.

CHEMICAL ATTACK / PEOPLE SUDDENLY FALLING ILL

– Leave the area of dispersal—do not walk through it—and go to the farthest car that you can reach.

– Remove outer clothing and rinse with copious amounts of water if you can.

– If unable to leave the train car, open windows.

– Do *not* activate the train's emergency brake, especially in a tunnel. Once the brake is pulled, the brakes have to be reset before the train can move again, thus increasing the time it takes for fire, police, and medical services to respond to incident. In addition, people will need to get to a station to receive specialized medical attention from emergency personnel. Use the emergency brake only when the forward motion of the train presents an imminent danger to life.

– For COMMUTER TRAINS, get off at the next station and leave the station.

– After exiting, if no one is there to assist you, remove outer clothing and find a place to wash off right away if you haven't already done so, then seek help from emergency responders.

BOMB OR EXPLOSION

– Move as far away from the explosion site as you can. Do not walk through the site if possible.

– Be extremely vigilant of your surroundings: terrorists may have a second bomb ready to detonate.

– If exiting through smoke, keep close to the ground and cover your mouth with fabric (wet if possible).

– Do *not* activate the emergency brake in the event of a fire or explosion, especially in a tunnel. Once the brake is pulled, the brakes have to be reset before the train can move again, thus increasing the time it takes for fire, police, and medical services to respond to the incident. Use the emergency brake only when the forward motion of the train presents an imminent danger to life.

EVACUATION

– Stay calm, and follow the instructions of the train crew.

– Do not take carry-on baggage with you—it will slow you and everybody else down.

- Climb over seats if the aisle is blocked.
- AMTRAK trains have windows equipped with emergency releases. Current models have a red handle at the top, which when pulled toward you and down, pulls the rubber seal off the window. The windowpane can then be pulled toward you from the top and removed.
- COMMUTER TRAINS with third-rail power: Don't attempt to leave the train on your own. In most circumstances, that's the most dangerous thing you can do. The third rail may still be electrified, and other trains may be in motion around you. The safest place for you is on the train unless instructed otherwise. If you can't stay in a car, walk calmly to another car that is unaffected by the emergency. Don't try to evacuate yourself from the train without help from the train crew or emergency personnel.
- For trains with catenary cables (overhead contact power lines), the above applies if the lines are down or near the ground.

Public Resources and Contact Information

GOVERNMENTAL AGENCIES FOR HEALTH AND EMERGENCIES

The American Veterinary Medical Association (AVMA) Veterinary Medical Assistance Team (VMAT) Program: Animal disaster preparedness and response
Website: *www.avma.org/vmat*
Animal and Plant Health Inspection Service (APHIS)
Website: *www.aphis.usda.gov*
Phone: 301-734-5267, Fax: 301-734-5941
FOIA Officer, 4700 River Road, Unit 50, Riverdale, MD 20737-1232
Centers for Disease Control and Prevention (CDC)
Website: *www.cdc.gov*
Bioterrorism Preparedness and Response Program: For public-health officials
    Phone: 770-488-7100
National Center for Environmental Health: For public-health officials
    24-Hour Emergency Telephone: 770-488-7100
National Immunization Hotline: 800-232-2522, *www.cdc.gov/nip*
Public Health Emergency Preparedness and Response
    Website: *www.bt.cdc.gov* (fact sheets on bioterrorism)
    Phone (directory): 404-639-3311
Public Response Hotline: For obtaining chemical/biological/
    radiological information—English Hotline: 888-246-2675,
    Spanish Hotline: 888-246-2857, TTY: 886-874-2646
    E-mail for questions: CDCresponse@ashastd.org
Environmental Protection Agency (EPA)
Website: *www.epa.gov/swercepp*
Phones: 800-424-9346, 703-412-9810, 800-553-7672 (TTY),
703-412-3323 (TTY)
Federal Bureau of Investigation (FBI) Operations Center
Website: *www.fbi.gov/terrorinfo/terrorism.htm*
Phone: 202-324-6700
Federal Disaster Medical Assistance Teams (DMATs)
Informational website: *www.hhs.gov/news/press/2001pres/20010911c.html*
Federal Emergency Management Agency (FEMA)
Website: *www.fema.gov*
Phone: 800-480-2520, 202-646-4600
    Citizen Preparedness Guide
        Website: *www.fema.gov/areyouready*
    FEMA Operations Center
        Phones: 800-634-7084, 540-665-6100, 703-771-6100
    FEMA National Preparedness Office
        Phone: 202-324-9025

Food Safety and Inspection Service (FSIS)
Website: *www.fsis.usda.gov* E-mail: fsis.webmaster@usda.gov
Phone: 202-690-3881, Fax: 202-690-3023
Food Safety and Inspection Service, United States Department of Agriculture
Washington, DC 20250-3700
Metropolitan Medical Strike Team (MMST)
Website: *ndms.dhhs.gov/CT_Program/MMRS/mmrs.html*
Metropolitan Medical Response System (MMRS)
Website: *www.mmrs.hhs.gov*
National Disaster Medical System (NDMS)
Website: *ndms.dhhs.gov/NDMS/ndms.html*
National Institutes of Health (NIH): Note, this is a research facility
and does not provide treatment
Website: *www.nih.gov*
Phone: 301-496-4000
Building 1, 1 Center Drive, Bethesda, MD 20892
National Pharmaceutical Stockpile (NPS): Part of the CDC
Website: *www.cdc.gov/nceh/nps/default.htm*
Phone: 404-639-0459
National Response Center: Chemical/biological/radiological hotline for
reporting incidents
Phone: 800-424-8802, 202-267-2675
Office of Emergency Preparedness (OEP): An office within the U.S.
Department of Health and Human Services
Website: *ndms.dhhs.gov* E-mail: ndms@usa.net
State public-health locator for officials, agencies, and public hotlines
Websites: *www.statepublichealth.org, www.cdc.gov/other.htm#states*
U.S. Army Medical Research Institute of Chemical Defense (USAMRICD)
Website: *ccc.apgea.army.mil*
Phone: 410-436-2230
Commander, USAMRICD, Attn: MCMR-UV-ZM
3100 Ricketts Point Road, Aberdeen Proving Ground, MD 21010-5400
U.S. Army Medical Research Institute of Infectious Diseases (USAMRIID)
Website: *www.usamriid.army.mil*
Response Line: 888-USA-RIID (888-872-7443)
Questions or Comments: USAMRIIDweb@amedd.army.mil
Commander, USAMRIID, Attn: MCMR-UIZ-R
1425 Porter Street, Fort Detrick, Frederick, MD 21702-5011
U.S. Department of Homeland Security
Website: *www.dhs.gov*
Homeland Security state contact list:
www.whitehouse.gov/homeland/contactmap.html

U.S. Department of Health and Human Services
Website: *www.hhs.gov*
Phone: 202-619-0257
U.S. Department of State: Terrorism-warning updates
Website: *www.state.gov*
U.S. Department of Transportation (DOT)
Website: *www.dot.gov* E-mail: dot.comments@ost.dot.gov
Phone: 202-366-4000
400 Seventh Street, SW; Washington, DC 20590
U.S. Food and Drug Administration (FDA)
Website: *www.fda.gov, www.fda.gov/oc/opacom/hottopics/bioterrorism.html*
Phone: 888-INFO-FDA (888-463-6332)
5600 Fishers Lane, Rockville MD 20857-0001

DISASTER RESPONSE AND RELIEF ORGANIZATIONS

American Red Cross National Headquarters
Website: *www.redcross.org*
Phone: 202-639-3520
431 Eighteenth Street, NW; Washington, DC 20006
AmeriCares Foundation
Website: *www.americares.org/splash.asp*
Phone: 800-486-HELP (800-486-4357)
161 Cherry Street, New Canaan, CT 06840
The Disaster Center
Website: *www.disastercenter.com/agency.htm*
Disaster Relief
Website: *www.disasterrelief.org*
The Salvation Army
Website: *www.salvationarmy.org*

INFORMATIONAL ONLINE RESOURCES

American Academy of Pediatrics: Children, Terrorism and Disasters
Website: *www.aap.org/terrorism/index.html*
American Medical Association
Website: *www.ama-asn.org*
American Psychological Association
Website: *helping.apa.org/daily/terrorism.html*
Apple Care Foundation: For information about ongoing research into new treatments, antidotes, and other medical and public safety programs related to emergent healthcare issues, including biological, chemical, and nuclear emergencies
Website: *www.applecarefoundation.org*
Association for Professionals in Infection Control and Epidemiology
Website: *www.apic.org/bioterror*

Center for Nonproliferation Studies (CNS), Monterey Institute for International Studies: Information on weapons of mass destruction
Website: *www.cns.miis.edu*

Center for the Study of Bioterrorism and Emerging Infections, St. Louis University
Website: *www.slu.edu/colleges/sph/bioterrorism/index.html*

Council on Foreign Relations, in cooperation with the Markle Foundation
Website: *www.terrorismanswers.com*

Federation of American Scientists
Website: *www.fas.org*

Infectious Diseases Society of America: Bioterrorism Information and Resources
Website: *www.idsociety.org/bt/toc.htm*

Johns Hopkins University Center for Civilian Biodefense Studies
Website: *www.hopkins-biodefense.org*
Phone: 410-223-1667

Medical NBC Online
Website: *www.nbc-med.org*

Medline-plus Health Information: A service of the National Library of Medicine and the National Institutes of Health
Website: *www.nlm.nih.gov/medlineplus/medlineplus.html*

The Survival Guide: What to Do in a Biological, Chemical, or Nuclear Emergency website: For updates, supplementary information, and helpful links
www.911guide.com

World Health Organization (WHO)
Website: *www.who.int/home-page*

PUBLICATIONS

Books

Weintraub, Pamela. *Bioterrorism: How to Survive the 25 Most Dangerous Biological Weapons.* Citadel Press, 2002.

Stilp, Richard, and Armando Bevelacque. *Citizen's Guide to Terrorism Preparedness.* Thomson-Delmar Learning, 2002.

Frist, Senator Bill. *When Every Moment Counts: What You Need to Know About Bioterrorism From the Senate's Only Doctor.* Rowman & Littlefield, 2002.

Articles

Bardi, Jason. "Aftermath of a hypothetical smallpox disaster," *Emerging Infectious Diseases,* vol. 5; 547–51 (August 1999).

Cieslak, Theodore J., and Edward M. Eitzen, Jr., "Clinical and epidemiologic principles of anthrax," *Emerging Infectious Diseases,* vol. 5; 552–5 (August 1999).

Centers for Disease Control and Prevention, "Management of patients with suspected viral hemorrhagic fever," *MMWR,* vol. 37 (S3); 1–16 (February 1988).

Henderson, D.A., "Smallpox: clinical and epidemiologic features," *Emerging Infectious Diseases,* vol. 5; 537–9 (August 1999).

Hugh-Jones, Martin E., "High-impact terrorism: proceedings from a Russian-American workshop," in *Agricultural Bioterrorism,* National Academies Press, 2002.

Journal of the American Medical Association (JAMA) series on biological weapons:

– Inglesby, Thomas V., *et al.* "Anthrax as a biological weapon: medical and public health management," vol. 281, no. 18 (May 1999).

– Arnon, Stephen S., *et al.* "Botulinum toxin as a biological weapon: medical and public health management," vol. 285, no. 8 (February 2001).

– Borio, Luciana, et al. "Hemorrhagic fever viruses as biological weapons: medical and public health management," vol. 287, no. 18 (May 2002).

– Inglesby, Thomas V., *et al.* "Plague as a biological weapon: medical and public health management," vol. 283, no. 17 (May 2000).

– Henderson, Donald A., *et al.* "Smallpox as a biological weapon: medical and public health management," vol. 281, no. 22 (June 1999).

– Dennis, David T., *et al.* "Tularemia as a biological weapon: medical and public health management," vol. 285, no. 21 (June 2001).

Khan, Ali S., and Michael J. Sage, in collaboration with the CDC Strategic Planning Workshop, "Biological and chemical terrorism: strategic plan for preparedness and response," Recommendations and Reports, *MMWR,* vol. 49 (RRO4); 1–14 (April 2000).

Meltzer, Martin I., *et al.*, "Modeling potential responses to smallpox as a bioterrorist weapon," *Emerging Infectious Diseases,* vol. 5; 959–69 (August 1999).

Mettler, Fred A., *et al.* "Major radiation exposure—what to expect and how to respond," *The New England Journal of Medicine,* vol. 346; 1554–6 (May 2002).

O'Toole, Tara, "Smallpox: an attack scenario," *Emerging Infectious Diseases,* vol. 5; 540–6 (August 1999).

Srinivasan, Arjun, "Glanders in a military research microbiologist," *The New England Journal of Medicine,* vol. 345; 256–8 (July 2001).

ONLINE PUBLICATIONS

American Academy of Pediatrics, "Family readiness kit: preparing to handle disasters," *www.aap.org/family/frk/frkit.htm,* 2003.

Batts-Osborne, Dahna, *et al.*, "Glanders and melioidosis," *eMedicine,* *www.emedicine.com/emerg/topic884.htm,* October 2001.

Chemical, Biological and Radiological (CBRN) Subcommittee, "Chemical/biological/radiological incident handbook," *www.cia.gov/cia/publications/cbr_handbook/cbrbook.htm,* October 1998.

Federal Emergency Management Agency and the American Red Cross, "Family disaster plan," *www.redcross.org/services/disaster/beprepared/fdp.pdf,* 2001.

Mirachi, Ferdinando L., and Michael Allswede, "Ricin," *eMedicine, www.emedicine.com/emerg/topic889.htm,* July 2002.

National Association of State Public Health Veterinarians (NSPHV), the American Veterinary Association, "Compendium of measures to control *Chlamydophila psittaci* (formerly *Chlamydia psittaci*) infection among humans (psittacosis) and pet birds," *www.avma/org/pubhlth/psittacosis.asp,* 2002.

U.S. Department of Justice, "United for a Stronger America: Citizens' Preparedness Guide," *www.ojp.usdoj.gov/ojpcorp/cpg.pdf*

PERSONAL EMERGENCY CONTACT INFORMATION

Doctor: _____

Area hospitals (addresses and numbers for information and emergency rooms; include as many as you can in your area):

_____

_____

_____

_____

Police Department: _____

Local poison control center: _____

Person and phone number of an out-of-state contact (in disasters, sometimes it is easier to get through on a long-distance call than locally):

_____

Person, address, and phone number of meeting place near your home in case of a sudden home emergency:

_____

_____

Person, address, and phone number of a distant meeting place in the event of an evacuation from your neighborhood:

_____

_____

E-mails of all family members and family contacts (sometimes E-mails can get through when calls cannot):

_____

_____

_____

Glossary

abscess – A localized collection of pus frequently surrounded by inflamed tissue; a cavity formed by the death and liquification of solid tissue.

acetylcholinesterase – An enzyme that breaks down acetylcholine, which is predominantly found in nerve endings to transmit nerve impulses. The action of this enzyme is inhibited by nerve agents.

acute – Refers to a health effect, usually of rapid onset and not prolonged; sometimes loosely used to mean "severe." Could also refer to brief exposure of high intensity.

aerosol – Liquid or solid particulate matter dispersed in air, gas, or vapor.

aerosolize – To process liquids or particles to make them airborne, as an aerosol.

agent – A factor such as a microorganism, chemical substance, or form of radiation that results in illness; something that is capable of producing an effect.

agroterrorism – The use of biological weapons against animals or crops.

air-purifying respirator – An air-filtering device that covers the nose and mouth (sometimes including an eye shield) and removes contaminants from the surrounding air by passing it through a filter, cartridge, or canister. A variety of filter cartridges are designed to capture specific particles and/or gases. Filters must be replaced once absorption capacity is depleted.

air-supplied respirator – A personal air-filtering device for long-term use that covers the face and uses a hose to deliver clean, safe air from a stationary source of compressed air. It is normally used when there are extended work periods required in atmospheres not immediately dangerous to life and health.

antibiotic – Strictly speaking, antibiotic means to inhibit or destroy life. Antibiotic drugs are soluble substances that inhibit the growth of other microorganisms.

antibodies – Found in the blood and body fluids of humans and animals, antibodies are proteins made by certain types of white blood cells. Specific antibodies are produced when the body is challenged by a specific foreign substance. Laboratory tests that identify the presence of specific antibodies to certain organisms indicate that the person has been exposed to the organisms that cause the disease.

antidote – A remedy that neutralizes poison or counteracts its effects. Antidotes are commonly used in the treatment of chemical-agent and other poisonous-substance exposure.

antitoxin – Antibodies (usually made from horse serum) that neutralize toxins, which are poisonous substances of biologic origin (such as toxins produced by bacteria).

antiviral – A drug that opposes a virus either by interfering with its replication or by weakening or abolishing its action.

asphyxiant – Any agent that interferes with respiration.

asphyxiation – The state of impaired or absent exchange of oxygen and carbon dioxide as would be necessary for normal breathing.

asymptomatic – Without symptoms or producing no symptoms of illness or disease.

atomic – Relating to an atom.

bacteria (plural of bacterium) – Any of a group of prokaryotic round, spiral, or rod-shaped single-celled microorganisms that usually multiply by cell division.

biological agent – A living organism or the material derived from it that causes disease in or harm to humans, animals, or plants, or causes deterioration of material. Biological agents may be used in the form of liquid droplets, aerosols, or dry powders.

blister agent – A substance that causes blistering of the skin.

blood agent – see *chemical asphyxiant*

bubo – The inflammatory swelling of a lymph gland (node); a characteristic finding in bubonic plague and other diseases causing lymph-node inflammation and enlargement.

cardiac – Pertaining to the heart.

CDC – see *Centers for Disease Control and Prevention*

Centers for Disease Control and Prevention (CDC) – Part of the U.S. Department of Health and Human Services and primarily located in Atlanta, Georgia, the CDC is the lead federal agency for protecting the health and safety of Americans, both at home and abroad. It provides information to medical professionals and the public to enhance health decisions. The CDC also develops and applies disease prevention and control, environmental health, health promotion, and educational activities designed to improve the health of the people of the United States.

central nervous system – The brain and spinal cord.

chemical agent – A chemical substance that is intended for use in military operations to kill, seriously injure, or incapacitate people through its physiological effects. Riot-control agents are not considered chemical agents.

chemical asphyxiant – A substance that injures a person by interfering with cell respiration (the exchange of oxygen and carbon dioxide between blood and tissues). Sometimes referred to as a "blood agent."

choking agent – see *pulmonary irritant*

chronic – Referring to a health-related state or condition that lasts a long time (the U.S. National Center for Health Statistics defines a chronic condition as one that lasts three months or longer) or recurs frequently; can also refer to prolonged or long-term exposure.

contagious – Capable of being transmitted from one organism to another; communicable or transmissible by contact with the sick or their fresh secretions or excretions.

culture – A population of microorganisms grown in a nutrient medium; used in order to identify the organism.

cutaneous – Relating to or affecting the skin.

decontamination – The process of making any person, object, or area safe by absorbing, destroying, neutralizing, making harmless, or removing a hazardous material.

defecation – To discharge feces from the rectum.

dehydration – Deprivation of water; the state of being low on bodily fluids. Signs are dark yellow, orangeish, and/or low volume of urine, low tear production, pale fingers, and wrinkled skin.

dermal – Relating to or affecting the dermis (skin).

dirty bomb – see *radiological dispersal device*

edema – An excessive accumulation of watery fluid in cells or tissues.

endemic – Belonging or native to a particular people, country, or locality; disease occurrence within a population that occurs with predictable regularity.

epidemic – An outbreak of disease; the occurrence in a community or region of cases of an illness or specific health-related event or behavior clearly in excess of normal expectancy.

FDA – see *U.S. Food and Drug Administration*

Federal Emergency Management Agency (FEMA) – The federal agency charged with building and supporting America's emergency management system. It is involved with the process through which emergency managers prepare for emergencies and disasters, respond to them when they occur, help people and institutions recover from them, mitigate their effects, reduce the risk of loss, and prevent disasters from occurring.

FEMA – see *Federal Emergency Management Agency*

gangrene – Tissue death (necrosis) due to obstruction, loss, or decrease of blood supply; it may be localized to a small area or involve an entire extremity (such as fingers or toes) or organ.

gas mask – A face covering or device used to protect the wearer from injurious gases and other noxious materials by filtering and purifying inhaled air. It usually consists of a face cover with two eyepieces and a mouthpiece that contacts a canister containing a filter; the filter absorbs noxious gases as they pass through the canister to the mouth. The face cover also has a one-way outlet valve for exhaled air.

gastrointestinal – Refers to both the stomach and intestines.

germicide – A substance that is destructive to germs and microbes.

groin – The area around the junction of the thigh and upper body.

half-life – The amount of time needed for half of the atoms of a radioactive material to decay (disintegrate).

hemorrhage – A copious discharge of blood from the blood vessels; to bleed.

HEPA (high-efficiency particle arresting) filters – Used in ventilation systems, HEPA filters were developed by the U.S. government to protect scientists from radioactive airborne particles. They remove 99.97% of particles 0.3 microns and smaller, which include dust, mold spores, dust mites, pet dander, allergens, and many biological agents such as anthrax spores. They do not purify the air of most chemical agents.

incapacitating agent – A substance that produces temporary physiological and/or mental effects via action on the central nervous system. Effects may persist for hours or days, but victims usually do not require medical treatment, though treatment may speed recovery.

infection – The entry and development of an infectious agent in the body of a person or animal. In an apparent "manifest" infection, the infected person outwardly appears to be sick. In an inapparent infection, there is no outward sign that an infectious agent has entered that person at all.

infectious – Capable of causing infection; a disease capable of being transmitted from person to person, with or without actual contact.

inhalation – The act of drawing in the breath.

intestinal tract – The digestive tube that passes from the stomach to the anus; it is divided primarily into the small and large intestines.

intravenous – Entering by way of a vein (i.e., through a needle).

ionize – To split off one or more electrons from an atom, thus leaving the atom with a positive electric charge; the electrons usually attach to one of the atoms or to molecules, giving them a negative charge.

ionizing radiation – Radiation that has sufficient energy to remove electrons from atoms; radiation that can cause injury to living tissues.

IV – Abbreviation for "intravenous."

jaundice – Yellow pigmentation of the skin and whites of the eyes (conjunctiva) caused by the deposition of bile pigments due to increased bile (bilirubin, the yellowish-brown or green fluid secreted by the liver) in the plasma.

latent – Dormant; not currently showing signs of activity or existence.

lesion – A wound or injury; an abnormal change in tissue due to injury or disease.

localized – Restricted to a definite part of the body; not general or systemic.

lymphatic system – A network of the body that includes the lymphatic vessels, lymph nodes, and tissues and is responsible for fighting infections and draining fluid from cells and tissues back to the bloodstream.

lymph gland – see *lymph node*

lymph node – One of numerous round, oval, or bean-shaped bodies located throughout the body along the course of lymphatic vessels, particularly in the neck, armpit, and groin areas. They contain numerous lymphocytes (a kind of white blood cell) that filter the flow of lymph fluid passing through the node. Sometimes referred to as "lymph glands."

malaise – A feeling of general discomfort or uneasiness, an "out-of-sorts" feeling; often the first indication of an infection or other disease.

meningitis – Inflammation of the meninges (membranes around the brain and spinal cord).

microorganism – An organism of microscopic or ultramicroscopic size.

mucous membranes – Moist membranes rich in glands that produce mucus; specifically, membranes that line body passages and cavities (e.g., eyes, mouth, lining of the throat and nasal passages) that communicate directly or indirectly with the exterior.

mucus – A gummy, slippery secretion produced by mucous membranes, which it moistens and protects.

mycotoxin – A toxic compound produced by fungi (molds).

nasal – Relating to the nose.

N95 respiratory mask – A disposable mask that covers the mouth and nose and filters air breathed in. The National Institute for Occupational Safety and Health (NIOSH) rates these masks according to how efficiently the filter blocks microscopic test particles of 0.3 microns in diameter; a rating of 95 means that at least 95% of particles that size are filtered out in tests (note that this means it does not completely eliminate exposure). The "N" means that the test was conducted with sodium chloride (NaCl) particles (in other filters, "P" signifies it is impenetrable by oils and "R" means it is resistant to oils).

National Pharmaceutical Stockpile (NPS) – The National Pharmaceutical Stockpile, part of the Centers for Disease Control, includes 12 collections of large emergency-response cargo containers placed strategically around the country. Called "push packs," they are filled with various medical supplies that can be delivered anywhere in the United States within 12 hours in the event of an emergency.

NBC suit – Outerwear for nuclear, biological, and chemical emergencies.

necrosis – Localized death of cells, tissues, or organs resulting from irreversible damage.

nerve agent – A chemical agent that interferes with the central nervous system.

neutralize – The rendering ineffective of any action, process, or substance; to counteract or make inert.

nuclear – Refers to radiation emanating from atomic nuclei or to atomic fission (as produced by a nuclear reaction).

nuclear reactor – A device in which a controlled, self-sustaining nuclear chain reaction can be maintained with the use of cooling to remove generated heat.

pandemic – Occurring over a wide geographic area and affecting an exceptionally high proportion of the population; a pandemic outbreak of a disease.

papule – A small, solid, circular bump on the skin.

paralysis – Complete or partial loss of function, especially when involving the movement in a muscle or sensation in a part of the body through injury or disease of the involved nerve supply.

pathogen – A specific agent—any virus, bacteria, or other substance—that causes disease.

pathogenic – Causing disease or abnormality.

persistent agent – A chemical agent that upon release retains its casualty-producing effects for an extended period, usually from 30 minutes to several days. It usually has a low evaporation rate and its vapor is heavier than air, hence its vapor cloud tends to be near the ground. It may be a long-term hazard. Although inhalation hazards are still a concern, extreme caution should also be taken to avoid skin contact.

petechiae – Reddish or purplish spots of pinpoint to pinhead size containing blood in the skin, which do not lose color with pressure; they can also form in mucous membranes.

phlegm – Mucus secreted in abnormally large quantity in the respiratory passages or mouth.

pneumonia – A disease of the lungs characterized by inflammation and solidification of formerly aerated tissue in which air spaces fill with fluid, immune-response cells, and fibrous proteins; caused by infection, irritants, or trauma.

pocket resuscitation mask – A device that protects a rescuer from being contaminated by a victim when giving emergency mouth-to-mouth resuscitation; it consists of a curved plastic cup that rests over a victim's mouth and has a short tube attached for the rescuer to blow into.

polymerase chain reaction (PCR) testing – A laboratory technique that uses DNA to help rapidly identify organisms.

powered air-purifying respirator (PAPR) – A motorized respirator system that uses a filter to clean surrounding air before delivered to the wearer to breathe; it typically includes a blower/battery box worn on the belt, headpiece, and breathing tube.

probiotics – The introduction of beneficial, naturally occurring bacteria into the body.

prophylaxis – Measures taken, such as pre-treatment even though infection has not been confirmed, designed to preserve health and prevent the spread of disease.

pulmonary – Relating to the lungs.

pulmonary irritant – A substance that causes physical injury to the lungs. In extreme cases, membranes swell and lungs become filled with fluid; death results from lack of oxygen. Sometimes referred to as a "choking agent."

push pack – A cargo container provided by the Centers for Disease Control that is filled with antibiotics, vaccines, antidotes, antitoxins, and other medical supplies that can be delivered anywhere in the United States within 12 hours in the event of a national medical emergency.

pustule – A small, circular bump on the skin, containing pus and having an inflamed base; it can resemble a blister or pimple.

quarantine – The isolation of a person with a known or possible contagious disease; it may be to a specially equipped medical facility. In extreme situations, it may be enforced.

radiation – High-energy particles or waves (e.g., alpha or beta particles or gamma rays) that are emitted by an atom as the substance undergoes radioactive decay.

radioactive decay – Loss of radioactivity with time; spontaneous emission of radiation or charged particles or both from an unstable nucleus. This process can be measured by using radiation detectors such as Geiger counters.

radioactive waste – Disposable, radioactive materials resulting from nuclear operations. Wastes are generally classified into two categories: high-level and low-level.

radiological dispersal device (RDD) – An explosive device (weapon or equipment) designed to disseminate radioactive material in order to cause destruction, damage, or injury by means of the radiation produced by the decay of such material; it does not involve a nuclear explosion. Also known as a "dirty bomb."

reference laboratory – A laboratory that will run medical tests ordered by doctors.

reservoir – Any person, animal, arthropod, plant, soil, or substance in which an infective agent normally lives and multiplies. The infectious agent primarily depends on the reservoir for its survival.

respiration – The act of breathing; the physical and chemical processes by which an organism supplies its cells and tissues with the oxygen needed for metabolism and relieves them of the carbon dioxide formed in energy-producing reactions.

respiratory – Relating to respiration.

respiratory failure – The loss of lung function, either acute or chronic, that results in subnormal oxygenation of blood or abnormally increased carbon dioxide; the inability to breathe by a person's own means.

self-contained breathing apparatus (SCBA) – A respiratory filter mask that contains its own air supply; it is composed of a face piece connected by a hose to a wearable, compressed, clean-air supply pack (like a scuba tank). Also called "supplied-air respirators."

sepsis – A toxic condition resulting from the spread of microorganisms or their toxins in the blood or tissues due to an infection; septicemia is a common type of sepsis.

septicemia – Systemwide disease, started from a localized infection, that is caused by the spread of microorganisms and their toxins via the circulating blood; formerly called "blood poisoning."

septic shock – Shock (inadequate blood flow and depleted oxygen to the cells) associated with infection and sepsis.

serology test – A blood test that measures specific antigens (something that causes an immune response) or antibodies formed due to invading infections using blood serum (the fluid portion of the blood).

shelter-in-place – In-place sheltering means protecting yourself inside where you are and staying there until given further instruction or the all-clear.

shock – A state characterized by inadequacy of blood flow throughout the body to the extent that damage occurs to cells and tissues; if prolonged, the cardiovascular system itself becomes damaged and begins to deteriorate, resulting in a vicious cycle that leads to death.

sodium hypochlorite – The active ingredient in household liquid chlorine bleach; it is ordinarily about 5% strength in a water-based solution of bleach.

spore – Some microorganisms, when nutritional resources are withdrawn, become inactive spores by forming hardy, protective shells around themselves; they are capable of converting to a reproductively viable organism when resources are restored, such as when they enter a human body.

sputum – Ejected matter made up of saliva, mucus, pus, and/or other discharges from the respiratory passages.

strain – A population of homogeneous organisms possessing a set of defined characteristics; regarding bacteria, a set of descendants that retains characteristics of its ancestor but differs from the original in some way.

supplied-air respirator – see *self-contained breathing apparatus (SCBA)*

supportive treatment – Treatment that involves no specific action against the agent causing illness but rather focuses on maintaining bodily functions. An example would be ventilator support for patients with breathing difficulties.

teratogenic – Causing abnormal development of an embryo or fetus.

third rail – A metal rail, usually running parallel to train tracks, through which electric current is led to the motors of a train or subway car; if it is electrified, touching it would cause severe shock or electrocution.

toxic – Poisonous; injurious to health or dangerous to life.

toxin – A poisonous substance formed during the metabolism and growth of certain living microorganisms (and some plants and animals); it is usually very unstable, notably toxic when introduced into the tissues, and typically capable of inducing antibody formation.

triage – A system of medical, emergency screening of patients (especially military or disaster victims) to determine their relative priority for treatment, with the purpose of maximizing the number of survivors.

U.S. Food and Drug Administration (FDA) – The purpose of the FDA is to promote and protect public health by helping safe and effective products—from common food ingredients to drugs to medical and surgical products—reach the market in a timely way and by monitoring products for continued safety.

vaccine – A preparation made from substances that would normally cause harm, such as viruses or bacteria (using pieces of them or killed or weakened organisms), that is administered in an inactive form to cause the body to make antibodies against them. Those antibodies will then protect a person if he or she is exposed to the active agent, such as the living virus or bacteria.

vapor – A substance in the gaseous state (as distinguished from the liquid or solid state).

vaporize – To convert a solid or liquid (such as by the application of heat or by spraying) into a vapor.

ventilation – Circulation of air; a system or means of providing fresh air.

ventilator – A device for maintaining artificial respiration; a breathing machine (also called a respirator).

viremia – Blood infection by a virus.

virulent – Extremely toxic and overcomes bodily defensive mechanisms; refers to a microorganism that causes severe disease.

virus – A group of infectious agents that, with few exceptions, are much smaller than most bacteria, are not visible through the light microscope, lack independent metabolism, and cannot grow or reproduce apart from living cells; they are regarded as extremely simple microorganisms or extremely complex molecules. Can also mean a disease caused by a virus.

volatile – Tending to evaporate rapidly, even at relatively low temperatures.

weaponize – To make something into a weapon; to enhance characteristics or to alter the spreadability of an agent to make it more weaponlike.

zoonosis – A disease that can be transmitted from animals to humans.

Acknowledgments

To my medical writer and researcher, Laurie A. Vandermolen, with whom I have greatly enjoyed working, your unfailing help, thoroughness, hard work, and dedication have made this book possible. To my friend Steven Hochberg, whose inspiration and enormous support led me to write this book, thank you. To my advisory board, Robert S. Hoffman, M.D., F.A.A.C.T., F.A.C.M.T., Evan T. Bell, M.D., Robert J. Barish, Ph.D., and Francis M. O'Hare, I thank you for your expertise and commitment to accuracy and for your invaluable recommendations toward public safety. I extend a special thanks to New York City Office of Emergency Management Commissioner, John T. Odermatt, whose friendship, enthusiasm, and assistance helped immensely in the writing of this book. I also thank Joshua D. Hartman, for pitching in with tenacity whenever we needed him, from computer assistance to emergency management consultation. To everyone else at the Ascent Group—particularly Bunny Ellerin, Allison Keeley, and Michael Feldman—thanks for all of your support and assistance. To my literary agent, Laura Dail, I offer my thanks for your vision and abiding determination to make the publishing of this book a reality. To Danielle Durkin at Random House, thank you for all of your efforts in shepherding this through to completion. Thanks also to our graphic designer, Cyndi Pena.

And finally, most important, to my loving, supportive family and most loyal, devoted friends. Throughout our lives, there are people who shape us, support us, encourage us, and allow us to realize our potentials and dreams; for me, these are my ever-present friends, V. A. Subramanian and William Hyman; my father and mother, Salvatore and Rosaria (Sara) Acquista; my brother and his wife, Dominick and Cathy Acquista, and their children, Salvatore, Dominick, and Sara.

Index

About the Author

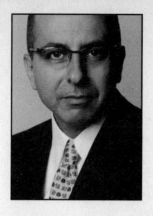

Angelo Acquista, M.D., received his medical degree at New York University School of Medicine in 1981 and is affiliated with Lenox Hill Hospital in Manhattan as an attending physician and clinical instructor in the Intensive Care Unit. He is board-certified in internal medicine, pulmonary medicine, and tropical diseases, and he is an Honorary Police Surgeon of the New York City Police Department. He also served on Mayor Rudolph Giuliani's Task Force on Bioterrorism and is the pro bono Medical Director for the New York City Office of Emergency Management. He also serves as Senior Medical Advisor for New York City Council Speaker Gifford Miller.

In addition, Dr. Acquista is a co-founder and co-chairman of the Apple Care Foundation, a not-for-profit organization dedicated to improving medical and public safety responsiveness to emergent healthcare issues. He is donating his proceeds from this book to the Foundation.

THE SURVIVAL GUIDE REFERENCE TABLE: What to Do in a Biological, Chemical, or Nuclear Emergency

EMERGENCY RESPONSE FOR BIOLOGICAL AGENTS: Leave the area of exposure immediately; cover your mouth and nose with fabric (wet if possible) or a respiratory mask; try not to breathe with out of out of exposure area; or take shallow breaths; make efforts to stay in place for decontamination by emergency personnel; seek shelter; wash body thoroughly with soap (rinse eyes and inside of mouth and nose with water); shower if possible; turn off ventilation systems such as air-conditioning, and close all doors, windows, and fireplace dampers; place exposed clothing and items in double plastic sealed bags; listen to TV or radio for emergency announcements; you may be instructed to shelter-in-place for a period of time; call your doctor if you think you have been exposed, especially if you begin developing any symptoms; do not begin treatment until instructed to do so.

	How You Get Exposed (Primarily)	Time from Exposure to Illness	Major Symptoms	Additional Emergency Responses (aerosol release)	Treatment	Vaccine
Anthrax	Inh, Ing, Skin	1-60 days	Flulike symptoms (fever, headache, abdominal pain, vomiting, coughing, chest pain) but no nasal congestion; increasingly severe breathing difficulties	Limit going from room to room, as this will spread anthrax spores around	Antibiotics	UD
Botulism	Inh, Ing	12-72 hours	Increasing muscle weakness and paralysis beginning in the face and progressing down the body symmetrically	If you are coming down with symptoms, go to a hospital (do not drive yourself)	Antitoxin	UD
Brucellosis	Inh, Ing, Skin; P-P unlikely but possible	2-3 weeks	Flulike symptoms, including fever; loss of appetite, cough, chest pain made worse by breathing		Antibiotics	N
Glanders and Melioidosis	Inh, Skin, MM, Anim; P-P rare but possible	Glanders: 10-14 days Melioidosis: Could be 2 days to years	Flulike symptoms including high fever, swollen neck glands, chest pain, congestion, pneumonia, open sores on mucous membranes and internal organs as well as a dark pink, pus-filled rash may develop	Hold eyes under running water for 15 minutes	Antibiotics	N
Pneumonic Plague	Inh; P-P	1-8 days	Fever, upset stomach, vomiting, diarrhea, muscle aches; then severe pneumonia-like symptoms with cough, chest pain, coughing up blood	Avoid outbreak area; use contact & respiratory precautions around infected persons; decontaminate exposed fabrics	Antibiotics	UD
Psittacosis	Inh; Bird or Anim; P-P likely rare	5-15 days	Fever, chills, sore throat, hacking cough, headache, muscle aches, pneumonia	Wash clothes in hot water	Antibiotics	N
Q Fever	Inh, Ing, Bug; P-P (rare)	14-40 days	Flulike symptoms including high fever, fatigue, weight loss, muscle pain, dry cough, sharp chest pain during inhalation, upset stomach, vomiting, diarrhea	Listen for instructions from emergency management personnel regarding environmental decontamination	Antibiotics	UD
Ricin	Inh, Ing, Injection	2-8 hours	Fever, chest tightness, cough, shortness of breath, nausea, joint pain, increasingly severe breathing difficulties	Wash body, clothes, and surfaces with soap and water and/or mild bleach solution	None, other than activated charcoal for ingestion	UD
Smallpox	Inh: Contact; P-P (highly contagious)	7-17 days	Flulike symptoms, including fever, vomiting, body aches, physical exhaustion, then deep, pus-filled bumps develop on face and limbs-less dense on torso; smallpox bumps all form and scab over at the same time	Avoid outbreak area; use contact & respiratory precautions around infected persons; decontaminate exposed fabrics; obtain vaccination immediately	Vaccination up to 4 days post-exposure, no treatment later	Y
Staphylococcal Enterotoxin B	Inh, Ing	3-12 hours	Fever, headache, chills, body aches, dry cough, shortness of breath, chest pain, could lead to severe breathing difficulties	Wash clothes in hot water	No specific treatment	UD
T2 Mycotoxin	Inh, Ing, Ab Skin and MM	Within minutes to 2-4 hours	Nasal pain, itching, and bleeding; sneezing; runny nose; mouth and throat pain; blood-tinged saliva; coughing; shortness of breath; wheezing; vomiting; hallucinations; skin burns and blistering	Take extra skin and eye precautions; gas mask is effective respiratory protection but not recommended to the untrained	None, other than activated charcoal for ingestion	UD
Tularemia	Inh, Ing, Skin, MM; Bug; Anim	1-21 days	Fever, muscle ache, malaise, sore throat, upset stomach, weakness, pneumonia with dry cough, sharp chest pain, rash, vomiting, diarrhea	Wash clothes with hot water	Antibiotics	UD
Viral Hemorrhagic Fevers (VHF)	Inh, MM; Contact; Bug; Anim	2-21 days	Fever; headache; muscle aches; extreme weakness; eye inflammation; rash; low blood pressure; bruising; bleeding from the eyes, mouth, ears, and/or rectum; kidney failure; confusion	Limit contact with infected persons; immediately wash any part of your body exposed to body fluids/excretions from suspected patients; take contact & respiratory precautions around patients; decontaminate objects or materials exposed to an infected person	For some, the antiviral drug ribavirin; for others, none	For yellow fever only

EMERGENCY RESPONSE FOR CHEMICAL AGENTS: Leave the exposure area immediately and seek fresh air-seconds may count; cover your mouth and nose with fabric (wet if possible); breathe as little as possible until out of exposure area or take shallow breaths; close eyes unless it inhibits escape; remove potentially exposed clothing and immediately rinse skin with copious amounts of water (shower if possible); even if symptom-free; flush eyes with water for 10-15 minutes; seek medical attention at once if you may have been exposed, as treatment should begin immediately; a gas mask or air-purifying respirator may be effective respiratory protection, but only recommended for trained professionals; listen to TV or radio for emergency announcements; be prepared to evacuate or shelter-in-place.

	How You Get Exposed	Time from Exposure to Illness	Major Symptoms	Additional Emergency Responses (aerosol release)	Treatment	Vaccine
Agent 15	Inh, Ing, Ab Skin	30 minutes to 36 hours	Dilated (widened) pupils, blurred vision, dry mouth and skin, illusions, hallucinations, denial of illness, impaired memory, short attention span		Antidote	—
Blister Agents	Inh, Ab Skin and MM (especially eyes)	Immediate to 2 days	Reddening, burning, itching of skin; large blister formation; eye and airway irritation; violent sneezing, sore throat; cough; chest pain; profuse mucus in nasal passages and airways; fluid-filled lungs; possible nausea and vomiting; PHOSGENE OXIME causes hives and welts versus large blisters	Close eyes unless it inhibits escape; do not go below ground level or lie on floor or ground as blister agents are heavier than air and will sink	Antidote for skin for lewisite; iodophors for skin	—
Chemical Asphyxiants	Inh and (less so) Ab Skin and eyes; Ing	Most immediate; ARSINE effects may be delayed for up to several hours	Irritation to eyes, nose, and airways; breathing difficulties; agitation; weakness; nausea; vomiting; muscular trembling; vertigo; violent convulsions; ARSINE causes red staining of the eyes, garlic breath odor; headache; thirst, shivering, weakness, jaundice, abdominal pain		Antidote kit (except for ARSINE)	—
Nerve Agents	Inh; MM; VX usually an oily liquid and Ab Skin	Seconds to minutes	Red, irritated, watery eyes; runny nose; sudden excess saliva/drooling; blood-tinged saliva and nasal secretions; shortness of breath; sweating; sneezing; dimmed or blurred vision; involuntary urination and/or defecation; vomiting; sudden loss of consciousness; seizure; paralysis	Do not go below ground level or lie on floor or ground; remain calm—it will benefit breathing ability; survival depends upon how quickly treatment is started and respiratory support given	Antidote	—
Pulmonary Irritants	Inh; Ab Skin and MM (especially eyes)	Usually rapid; effects of CHLORINE may be delayed	Burning eyes and throat, chest pain and tightness, chest pain, shortness of breath; life-threatening fluid-filled lungs may follow, indicated by severe shortness of breath and frothy saliva coming from mouth and/or nose	Close eyes unless it inhibits escape; do not go below ground level or lie on floor ground, remain calm—it will benefit breathing ability	No specific treatment	—

EMERGENCY RESPONSE FOR RADIATION EXPOSURE: If potentially exposed, the basic ways to protect yourself are through **(1) Time**—decreasing the time spent exposed to the radiation source; **(2) Distance**—getting as far away as possible from the source; and **(3) Shielding**—Seeking shelter and creating as thick a barrier as possible between you and the radiation; even clothing and glass can shield from some types of radiation. Go to a basement without windows if possible or inner room; wash thoroughly with soap and water (shower if possible); you may be directed to a decontamination site; turn off ventilation systems; a gas mask may be effective respiratory protection, but only recommended for trained professionals; listen to TV or radio for emergency announcements; be prepared to evacuate or shelter-in-place for several days or more.

	How You Get Exposed	Time from Exposure to Illness	Major Symptoms	Additional Emergency Responses (aerosol release)	Treatment	Vaccine
Dirty Bombs Nuclear	Inh, Ing, Ab Skin	Minutes to years; most injuries due to explosion itself	Acute radiation poisoning extremely unlikely after dirty-bomb detonation; for signs of severe exposure, see **nuclear bomb**	Leave the immediate area on foot; avoid mass transit; note that KI treatment not likely necessary	Potassium iodide (KI)	—
Nuclear Bombs and Nuclear Reactors	Inh, Ing, Ab Skin	Minutes to years	Signs of severe radiation exposure include burning of skin with redness, blistering, and peeling; inflammation of skin and mucous membranes; dehydration; nausea; vomiting; diarrhea; convulsions; exhaustion. Delayed symptoms include open sores on skin and in mouth or along intestinal tract; bloody diarrhea, or vomit, bleeding from the nose, mouth, and gums; bruising; and hair loss	For nuclear bomb, don't look directly at detonation as it could cause permanent eye damage; take KI if radioactive iodine is confirmed (see chapters for risks associated with it)	Potassium iodide (KI)	—

Inh = Inhaled; Ing = Ingested, Skin = Through break in the skin, Ab Skin = Absorbed into the skin, MM = Through mucous membranes, Contact = Direct patient contact, including secretions and clothing, Bug = Insect bite, Anim = Animal contact, P-P = Person-to-person transmission; Y = Yes, N = No, UD = Under development

IMPORTANT PHONE NUMBERS: CDC Information Hotline: 888-246-2675; CDC Immunization Hotline: 800-232-2522; National Response Center, Chemical/Biological/Radiological Hotline for reporting incidents: 800-424-8802
IMPORTANT WEBSITES: Federal Emergency Management Agency (FEMA): *www.fema.gov* State public-health locators for officials, agencies, and public hotlines: *www.statepublichealth.org* and *www.cdc.gov/other.htm#states*
U.S. Department of Homeland Security: *www.dhs.gov* State contact list: *www.whitehouse.gov/homeland/contactmap.html*